Reforming Long-term Care in Europe

D1516013

Broadening Perspectives on Social Policy
Series Editor: Bent Greve

The object of this series, in this age of re-thinking on social welfare, is to bring fresh points of view and to attract fresh audiences to the mainstream of social policy debate.

The choice of themes is designed to feature issues of major interest and concern, such as are already stretching the boundaries of social policy.

This is the fourteenth collection of papers in the series. Previous volumes include:

Reforming Long-term Care in Europe

Edited by

Joan Costa-Font

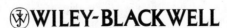

A John Wiley & Sons, Inc., Publication

This edition first published 2011
Originally published as Volume 44, Issue 4 of *Social Policy & Administration*
Chapters © 2011 The Authors
Book compilation © 2011 Blackwell Publishing Ltd

Blackwell Publishing was acquired by John Wiley & Sons in February 2007.
Blackwell's publishing program has been merged with Wiley's global Scientific,
Technical, and Medical business to form Wiley-Blackwell.

Registered Office
John Wiley & Sons Ltd, The Atrium, Southern Gate, Chichester, West Sussex,
PO19 8SQ, United Kingdom

Editorial Offices
350 Main Street, Malden, MA 02148-5020, USA
9600 Garsington Road, Oxford, OX4 2DQ, UK
The Atrium, Southern Gate, Chichester, West Sussex, PO19 8SQ, UK

For details of our global editorial offices, for customer services, and for information
about how to apply for permission to reuse the copyright material in this book
please see our website at www.wiley.com/wiley-blackwell.

The right of Joan Costa-Font to be identified as the author of the editorial
material in this work has been asserted in accordance with the UK Copyright,
Designs and Patents Act 1988.

Library of Congress Cataloging-in-Publication Data

Reforming long-term care in Europe / edited by Joan Costa-Font.
 p. cm. – (Broadening perspectives in social policy ; 6)
 Includes bibliographical references and index.
 ISBN 978-1-4443-3873-7 (pbk.)
 1. Older people–Long-term care–Government policy–Europe. 2. Older people–
Europe–Social conditions. 3. Older people–Government policy–Europe. I. Costa-
Font, Joan.
 HV1481.E782R44 2011
 362.16094–dc22

2011001477

A catalogue record for this book is available from the British Library.

Set in 10.5 on 11 pt Baskerville MT by Toppan Best-set Premedia Limited
Printed in Malaysia by Ho Printing (M) Sdn Bhd

1   2011

CONTENTS

Editorial Introduction

Joan Costa-Font

Welcome to this book on European long-term care reform. Hopefully, you will find a very relevant set of chapters that we expect will influence the scholarly and policy debates on how best to reform the financing and organization of long-term care in Europe.

All contributors to this book have focused on an issue regarding the reform of long-term care (LTC) in their specific country of study. That is, they attempt to explain reforms in LTC provision and financing by focusing on a central issue in the social policy debate in their countries. The central theme has been left to the author's choice, and the aspects discussed in each country are arguably a good picture of the most relevant country-specific policy questions. Furthermore, the country case studies under analysis have been selected on the basis of the existing (or lack of) evidence on the ongoing reforms in each country, and the existing literature about it. For instance, very little has been written so far on LTC reform in Eastern European countries, and almost no research is available on the reasons for reform or non-reform of LTC in Southern Europe. It was perceived that more research should be done on the sustainability of LTC financing in established systems such as the Dutch one, and on the reforms in France.

The chapters you will find in this book can be divided into two sections. The first section contains six chapters dealing with reforms in the financing of long-term care, and includes conceptual contributions alongside empirical studies from different countries in Europe, including reforms in the UK, the Netherlands, France, Germany and Eastern Europe. Then a second section looks at contributions on the reform of the organization of LTC in Spain, Italy, Sweden and Portugal.

The first chapter, by Nicholas Barr, provides an overview of traditional claims in favour of social insurance as a means of funding LTC. In particular, it examines its economic rationale and highlights that an entitlement to care is made clear in the event of old-age dependency. The second chapter, by Adelina Comas-Herrera, Raphael Wittenberg and Linda Pickard, contains an examination of policy developments in reforming LTC in the UK. It describes the rationale for reform in Britain, drawing upon the evidence of the Royal Commission and the institutional and policy designs that explore the role of choice and the provision of care. This chapter is followed by a chapter by Blanche Le Bihan and Claude Martin that examines the policy discussions that have grounded reform of LTC in France. Next, the experience of financial reform and stability of the financing of LTC in the Netherlands is evaluated in a chapter by Frederik T. Schut and Bernard van den Berg. As an example of a system of social insurance, the following chapter, by Heinz Rothgang, provides an analysis of the reforms in financing of LTC in Germany. This section is completed with a final chapter by August Österle that explores financing reforms in Central and South-Eastern Europe, where evidence from seven countries is reported: Croatia, the Czech Republic, Hungary, Romania, Serbia, Slovakia and Slovenia.

The second section discusses reforms in the organization of long-term care. This section contains three chapters. The first, authored by myself, examines the political economy of long-term care reform (and absence of reform) in Italy and Spain; I draw specifically upon the influence devolution played as a source of reform and fragmentation in Spain, and against reform in Italy. Next, reform and the question of the local variability of LTC services in Sweden is discussed by Gun-Britt Trydegård and Mats Thorslund. The final chapter is by Silvina Santana, and deals with the formal and informal settings of LTC in Portugal, focusing on two aspects: service quality and problems with the organization of care, which are essential in understanding developments in Portugal.

This book would not have been possible without the enthusiastic reception by the editorial committee of the journal, and particularly Bent Greve, and the always altruistic help of anonymous referees, which we acknowledge here. Particularly, we wish to thank Cristiano Gori, Bleddyn Davies, Andreas Hoff, Guillem Lopez Casasnovas, Ana Guillén, Anna Maria Simonazzi, Birgit Trukeschitz, Martin Powell, Martin Karlsson, Carla Rodríguez, Jolanta Aidukaite, Lucia Kosarova, Jérôme Wittwer, Christophe Courbage, Javier Hernandez, Gerdt Sundström and Francesca Bettio. Some chapters did not make it into the book due to our tight timing and our quality constraints, but as usual we hope that the motivation of participating in the book was an incentive to improve and/or complete them. Finally, I hope you enjoy reading this book as much as we enjoyed preparing it.

1

Long-term Care: A Suitable Case for Social Insurance

Nicholas Barr

The Backdrop

This chapter discusses the finance of long-term care (LTC), including care in a person's own home (domiciliary care) and residential care, including nursing care. I argue that there are welfare gains from being able to insure LTC expenditures, but the mechanism of actuarial insurance is not well suited to the risks associated with needing long-term care.

The remainder of this section explains why the ability to insure is beneficial and how the actuarial mechanism works. The next two sections discuss in turn the technical problems facing providers of long-term care insurance and the information problems facing individuals looking to buy such insurance, that is, problems on both supply and demand sides of the insurance market. The following section considers a range of solutions, including finance from general taxation and social insurance. The final section offers some strategic conclusions.

Why insurance?

In the right circumstances, insurance has powerful advantages, both in efficiency terms and from a moral perspective.

Efficiency arguments. To illustrate the potential welfare gains from insurance, assume that high-quality long-term care costs €30,000 per year, that one in six people needs long-term care and, if so, needs it on average for two years. Thus the typical person needs long-term care for one-third of a year, at a cost of €10,000.

In principle, there are two ways in which a person could seek to finance such costs.

- Actuarial insurance: if it is possible to buy insurance at an actuarially fair price (and ignoring transaction costs), a person has to save enough to cover the *average* duration, e.g. one-third of a year = €10,000.

- Self-insurance: in a world with no insurance, a person who seeks security must save enough to cover the *maximum* potential duration of long-term care, e.g. 20 years at €30,000 per year = €600,000.

Thus the welfare gains from insurance are large and obvious: a person who is risk-averse does not have to set aside €600,000, but instead pays insurance premiums which (in present value terms) total €10,000. A core conclusion is that insurance dominates self-insurance.

Moral arguments. The philosopher John Rawls (1972) argues that in a just society the rules are made by people who do not know where they will end up in that society, that is, they are made behind what he called the Veil of Ignorance. Insurance can be interpreted as an example of solidarity behind the Veil of Ignorance: a person who joins a risk pool does not know in advance whether or not he will suffer a loss and hence have to make a claim. Insurance thus has moral appeal.

How actuarial insurance works

The easiest way to see how actuarial insurance works is by example. Suppose that there are 100 of us, that we decide to fly to Rome to see a football match, that each of us has a suitcase worth €1,000, and that on average 2 per cent of suitcases get lost. Thus each of us faces a potential loss, L, of €1,000, which occurs with a probability, p, of 2 per cent. In those circumstances, it would be possible to collect 2% × €1,000 = €20 from each of the 100 people, i.e. €2,000 in total; in Rome, we would find which two people had lost their suitcase, and pay each €1,000 in compensation.

More formally, the actuarial premium for the ith individual, π_i, is defined as:

$$\Pi_i = (1+a)\, p_i L \tag{1}$$

where $p_i L$ is the individual's expected loss, and α is the loading the insurance company charges to cover administrative costs and competitive profit; π is the price at which insurance will be supplied in a competitive market. For the purposes of this chapter, insurance is actuarial if, as in equation (1), the premium is based on the risk of an event occurring and the size of the resulting loss.

The intuition of this mechanism is straightforward. Insurance premiums are high where the probability of loss is high (a young car driver) or where the potential size of the loss is large (driving a Rolls Royce).

This, broadly, is the way in which actuarial insurance operates. Thus far there is no need for state intervention. A rational risk-averse person facing a known risk will buy insurance, which the market can and will supply.

Problems for Insurers

Technical problems on the supply side

Insurance along the lines of equation (1) is efficient only if a number of conditions hold. Where they fail, actuarial insurance may be inefficient or impossible.

Individual risk, not common shock. Insurance requires that the probabilities in equation (1) are independent, that is, that there are a predictable number of winners and losers. This applies to car accidents (if I crash my car, this does not affect the likelihood that you will crash your car). With a common shock, in contrast, if one person suffers a loss, so does everyone else. If I suffer 5 per cent inflation this year so, broadly, does everyone else. Actuarial insurance generally cannot cope with common shocks.

Risk, not certainty. Insurance is a device to accommodate risk. Thus p_i in equation (1) must be less than one. If $p_i = 1$, it is certain that the insured person's car will be stolen, and the insurance premium will exceed the insured loss. There is no possibility of spreading risks, hence no gain from joining a risk pool. The problem arises in two ways with medical insurance. First is old age: the probability of elderly people requiring medical care is high. A separate problem is pre-existing medical conditions: actuarial insurance can cover *potential* problems, but not *actual* problems, that is, medical problems which the individual already has at the time that he/she applies for insurance. Pre-existing medical conditions are generally uninsurable.

The two conditions just discussed relate to the fundamental nature of insurance as a device for sharing risk. The remaining conditions reflect information problems in insurance markets.

Risk, not uncertainty. The insurer needs to estimate p_i in equation (1) with reasonable precision in order to calculate a premium. Insurance can cope with risk (where the probability is known) but not with uncertainty (where it is not).[1] There are various circumstances in which the probability might not be well known.

- Where the insured event is rare (e.g. early satellite launches), estimates of the probability will have a large variance.
- Where the problem is complex. Actuarial insurance against future inflation is impossible because the probability of different levels of future price increases cannot be predicted.[2]
- Where the insured event has a long time horizon.

A further condition is that all participants – both buyer and seller of insurance – must be equally well informed. The failure of this condition – asymmetric information – creates two further potential problems: adverse selection and moral hazard.

Adverse selection. Efficient insurance requires that high-risk individuals pay a premium calculated from equation (1), based on a high probability of loss, P_H, and low-risk individuals pay a premium based on their low probability, p_L. With automobile insurance, someone who is twice as risky pays roughly twice the insurance premium.

Adverse selection arises where the buyer can conceal from the insurer the fact that he is a bad risk, and is thus an insurance-market manifestation of 'lemons' (Akerlof 1970). The problem is not that people differ in their riskiness, but that the insurer is less well-informed than the buyer about the applicant's riskiness. The individual knows he is a 'lemon' (i.e. a bad risk), but can conceal the fact from the insurer, hence the description of adverse selection as 'hidden knowledge'. The problem can arise if health care is an important part of employer benefits: firms with the best health-care packages will tend to attract workers with health problems, thus reducing the firm's competitiveness.

Moral hazard. A second class of asymmetric information, moral hazard, arises where the insured person can influence the insurer's expected loss, p_iL in equation (1), without the insurer's knowledge (hence moral hazard is sometimes described as 'hidden action'). The problem arises in two ways, concerning p_i and L, respectively.

1. *Endogenous probability*: here individuals can manipulate the probability of the insured event at little or no cost to themselves. If people are insured they might drive less carefully. My extra spending on maintaining the brakes on my car reduces the probability that I will have an accident. But the insurer cannot monitor such expenditure and so will reduce my premium not by the (significant) decline in the probability that I will have an accident but by the (much smaller) decline averaged across all the drivers it insures. Thus the main beneficiaries of my spending on safety are other insured people who now pay slightly lower premiums. Given this externality, individuals face incentives to underinvest in preventive activities. Moral hazard causes inefficiency, since people take less care than if they had to bear the full loss themselves.

   A second manifestation of endogenous probability arises where insurance is concerned not with an undesirable event that is beyond the individual's control but with a desirable event that the individual can choose, the standard example being voluntary pregnancy. Individuals face no psychic cost, and can control the probability, p_i, in equation (1). This situation is very different from an unwelcome exogenous event – the problem insurance is meant to address. Cases of this sort are generally uninsurable for individuals.[3]

2. *Endogenous L* (the 'third-party payment problem'): here the individual can influence the size of the insured loss, L. The intuition is straightforward – contrast the amount of champagne people drink if they pay for it themselves with their consumption of champagne provided free by the airline. Similarly, if the insurer pays all medical costs, both doctor and patient can act as though health care were free, even though its social cost is positive, and generally large. Moral hazard in this form leads to inefficiently high spending.

The problem of moral hazard is fundamental: the more complete the cover and the lower the psychic loss from the insured event, the less individuals have to bear the consequences of their actions and the less, therefore, the incentive to behave as they would if they had to bear their losses themselves.

One way of seeking to reduce the problem is through inspection of damage before meeting a claim, for example with automobile repairs. An alternative is to use incentive mechanisms, by sharing the cost between the individual and the insurer: frequent claimants (e.g. accident-prone car drivers) pay higher premiums; deductibles require the insured person to pay the first €X of any claim, coinsurance to pay the first x per cent. None of these approaches, however, faces the individual with the full marginal cost of any loss.

In analytical terms, adverse selection and moral hazard are both examples of imperfect information. If the insurer could read the thoughts of insurees there could be no hidden knowledge or hidden action.

Problems with long-term care insurance

When considering long-term care insurance it is helpful to distinguish two probabilities:

- p_1 is the probability that a person will need care at some stage in his/her life;
- p_2 is the probability distribution, *given that a person needs care*, of different durations of that care.[4] If we assume that once someone needs care they will do so for the rest of their life this probability equals remaining life expectancy at the time a person first needs care.

When applied to long-term care, equation (1) becomes:

$$\Pi_i = (1+a)\,p_{1i}L(p_{2i}) \tag{2}$$

where p_{1i} is the probability that the ith person will need long-term care at some stage, and $L(p_{2i})$ is the cost of care conditional on the person's remaining life expectancy at the date he or she first needs care.

To what extent does long-term care conform – or fail to conform – with the conditions in the previous section?

Independence. Probabilities of needing long-term care may not be independent. If a medical advance prolongs life to the point where more people end up needing care (i.e. an increase in p_1), the result is to increase the probability of needing long-term care for *all* policy-holders. This outcome would arise, for example, with dramatic progress in addressing cardiovascular disease and cancer, but much less in addressing dementia, since more people would live to ages where dementia arises. Similar issues can arise with p_2, for example, a medical advance that increases the average life expectancy of people in care.

Uncertainty. This is a problem for both (a) the relevant probabilities and (b) the costs of care. Each requires discussion.

Case 1: buying insurance when young. Let us start with a young person wanting to buy insurance. Insurers have a broad idea of p_1 and p_2 for today's frail elderly. What they need to know, however, are the relevant probability distributions for *future* cohorts.

Over the medium term, neither probability is known, since each can change over a long time horizon (a person aged 30 buys a policy under which he might not make a claim for 60 years).

- p_1 might get smaller because medical advances help people to care for themselves (e.g. tablets that deal with arthritis) or because of technical advances with the same effect (e.g. cheap robots doing household chores for housebound arthritics). On the other hand, medical progress, by extending life, might increase the likelihood of requiring care.
- p_2 might get smaller because medical advances keep people out of care for longer, so that remaining average life expectancy at the time care starts is less. On the other hand, if medical progress extends the duration of dependent life, the probability might increase.

Thus the relevant probabilities cannot be known far in advance, and even the direction of change is unknown. Over such a long time horizon, the issue becomes one of uncertainty rather than risk.

Case 2: buying insurance at the time a person needs care. There is a tension between encouraging people to buy a policy at a younger or an older age. With younger people, the range of uncertainty facing the insurer is greater but so are the gains to the individual from risk-pooling. With older people, uncertainty is less but, since some people now have a high probability of requiring care, the opportunity of risk-pooling is reduced.

The limiting case arises where a person takes out insurance only when he/she needs care. In this case, there is no uncertainty about p_1, which equals one. Nor is there a major problem about p_2 which, at its simplest, is the person's remaining life expectancy, that is, his/her longevity risk. In this case, long-term care insurance is equivalent to buying an annuity that pays €X per year for the rest of a person's life, where €X is the annual cost of care.

How do the two cases compare? Let us return to the earlier example, where care costs €30,000 per year and one in six people needs long-term care and, if so, needs it on average for two years. Thus, ignoring transaction costs:

- Buying insurance when young: if the probabilities are known, a representative person needs care for one-third of a year, and so can buy insurance for €10,000, i.e. one-third of €30,000.
- Buying insurance when care is first needed: a person entering long-term care typically needs it for two years, so that the relevant annuity costs €60,000, i.e. two years at €30,000 per year. A deferred annuity (e.g. one that pays for care only after the first two years, but thereafter for life) would be cheaper because insurance cover is only partial.
- With no insurance, the person has to save for (say) 20 years, i.e. €600,000. This is true whether we are talking about simple private savings or such devices as a long-term care savings account, and whether or not there are tax incentives towards such saving activities.[5]

In comparing these options, the welfare rankings are clear: Case 1 is superior to case 2, which is superior to no insurance. Wider risk-pooling dominates narrower risk-pooling; and insurance dominates self-insurance.

Thus far we have discussed uncertainty about p_1 and p_2. Uncertainty about the annual cost of care, L, is a separate problem. It is well known that the relative cost of services rises over time.[6] But over the long term, the ability to predict the costs of care becomes questionable. Will costs rise because the cost of skilled labour rises? Or will expensive labour be partially replaced by cheaper capital (e.g. robots for some tasks) or by cheaper pharmaceutical drugs? As with uncertainty about the relevant probabilities, there is doubt even about the direction of change.

For both reasons – uncertainty about the probabilities and about costs – there is a considerable 'funnel of doubt' about total future spending on long-term care. The UK Royal Commission's sensitivity tests suggest that the total could vary by a factor of two (£21 billion to £39 billion) in 2031, and by a factor of nearly three (£28 billion to £76 billion) in 2051 (UK Royal Commission 1999: table 5.1; see also Nuttall *et al.* 1995). In the face of such uncertainty, voluntary private insurance becomes highly problematical.

Adverse selection. As with medical insurance, the person buying insurance, knowing that s/he is a bad risk, might be able to conceal that fact from the insurer. Irrespective of reality, the efficiency of insurance markets suffers when insurers *think* adverse selection is a reality. Evidence from the USA (Sloan and Norton 1997) suggests that adverse selection, whether real or perceived, is a problem.

Moral hazard. This arises in two ways. A person who has insurance that covers all the costs of long-term care is more likely to demand care since the cost to him or her (at the time of use) is zero. This is the third-party payment problem familiar from medical insurance. There is an extensive literature on the range of instruments – incentive or regulatory – that seek to contain costs in such circumstances.

Incentive-based mechanisms to contain spending include:

- cost-sharing via deductibles (where the individual pays the first €X per year) or co-payments (where the individual pays x per cent of the costs);
- preferred providers, whereby suppliers are chosen on the basis of competitive bidding;
- prospective payment mechanisms like health maintenance organizations or diagnosis-related groups.[7]

Regulation of spending includes:

- controlling the price that providers can charge;
- imposing an annual budget cap. This can take the form of a global annual budget for a hospital. Or the cap can be at the level of the individual physician. Or the cap can be on reimbursement of all physicians, for

example by retrospectively reducing agreed fees if physicians prescribe a greater volume of treatment than planned.

Long-term care faces most of these problems. In particular, if the insurance company pays all the costs, a person is more likely to request care and/or to request luxurious accommodation.

In contrast, a second aspect of moral hazard is very different from medical care. The third-party incentive increases the likelihood that a person will demand care. But in this case, the incentive applies not only to the policy-holder but also to his or her family. Insurance cover changes the balance of probability between care from family members and care by others. To guard against being put into residential care against one's will, it could therefore be rational not to insure (Pauly 1990; Sloan and Norton 1997).

Thus insurers are imperfectly informed, and so design policies which reduce their exposure to risk in several ways. To guard against uncertainty, premiums err on the side of safety. There is a cap on the total payout per year (though not usually on the number of years), thus limiting L in equation (2). Insurers attempt to counter adverse selection by requiring full disclosure of an applicant's medical history, where a failure to disclose a 'relevant' fact invalidates the policy even where the insurer has not specifically asked for the fact. Attempts to guard against moral hazard include contracts which offer cover against tightly-defined criteria, rather than for a more general need for care.

Problems for Individuals

Alongside these supply-side problems are problems from the perspective of individuals. Insurance policies for long-term care are both long-term and complex. As a result, consumers face many of the problems now widely recognized from the economics of information and behavioural economics. The following questions illustrate the problems individuals face in choosing an insurance policy in a competitive system.

What type of care is covered? Does the policy cover only residential care, or also domiciliary care; is a person entitled to residential care on the basis of general infirmity or only if he or she has clearly defined, specific ailments? How will the answers to these questions change with advances over the years in medical technology?

On what financial basis is care provided? Can the insurer increase premiums if a person becomes more risky (i.e. if p_1 or p_2 rises); is there a ceiling on the monthly cost of care; is there a maximum duration over which benefit is payable? Will those figures change over time in line with changes in prices, changes in wages, or changes in the cost of care?

How well specified is the contract? Can insurers change the basis of cover; does the wording make clear the circumstances in which an individual can make choices; what arrangements deal with any disagreements between the policy-holder and the insurer?

Complications arise, further, because people may not know how much cover they actually have. If public funding becomes more generous, people with extensive private insurance end up with an inefficiently large amount of cover. Conversely, cuts in public funding may leave people under-insured; and if such under-insurance occurs relatively late in life, additional private cover is expensive.

In the face of such complexities, Burchardt and Hills (1997: ch. 6) found that even their academic study could not unearth the data necessary for proper assessment of policies, calling seriously into question the ability of individuals to make informed choices. At a minimum, there is need for regulation to ensure that all policies cover at least a basic package.

Strategic Policy Directions

Private, actuarial insurance works well for risks that conform with the conditions discussed earlier, for example, automobile insurance and burglary insurance. But that does not mean that the mechanism can be applied uncritically to other areas. The conclusion of earlier discussion is that the mechanism faces major technical problems when applied to long-term care. Given the range of problems facing both sides of the market, the conclusion of the UK Royal Commission on Long Term Care (1999: 93), should not be surprising:

> Left to grow without intervention, there seems little reason to think that private insurance will become more important in the UK than it has become . . . in America. At present only 4%–5% of Americans have taken out long-term care insurance, while 10%–20% could afford to do so and 80%–90% could not afford the cost in any event.

Social insurance as a response to information problems

In his classic article, Kenneth Arrow (1963) argues that, where markets fail, other institutions may arise to mitigate the resulting problems: 'the failure of the market to insure against uncertainties has created many social institutions in which the usual assumptions of the market are to some extent contradicted' (1963: 967). This line of argument contrasts with that of Hayek (1945). Both Arrow and Hayek started from the assumption of asymmetric information. To Hayek the fact that different people know different things is an argument *in favour* of markets. He argued that (as with skill differences) the market makes beneficial use of such differences by allowing gains from trade.

Arrow shows that the market is an inefficient device for mediating certain important classes of differences in knowledge between people. Nor is his view idiosyncratic. When discussing unemployment, Lucas (1987: 62) reached an identical conclusion:

> Since . . . with private information, competitively determined arrangements will fall short of complete pooling, this class of models also raises the issue of *social insurance*: pooling arrangements that are not actuarially sound, and hence require support from compulsory taxation. The main

elements of Kenneth Arrow's analysis of medical insurance are readily transferable to this employment context. (emphasis in original)

Social insurance thus derives from two sources. The need for insurance arises because, at least in Western countries, the risk of needing long-term care is to some extent a social construct (the greater the fragmentation of extended families and the more widespread women's labour-market activity, the greater the likelihood that family support for the frail elderly will be insufficient).[8] Second, on the supply side, information failures and the inability of actuarial insurance to address common shocks provide both a theoretical justification of and an explanation for institutions such as social insurance.

Conventional social insurance mimics private institutions: benefits are conditioned on an implicit or explicit contributions record and on the occurrence of a specified event such as reaching pensionable age. Administration can be by the state at national or subnational level; or administration can be hived off to institutions such as friendly societies or trades unions.

Social insurance, however, differs from private insurance in two important respects. First, because membership is generally compulsory, it is *possible* (though not essential) to break the link between premium and individual risk. Second, the contract is usually less specific than private insurance, with two advantages: protection can be given against risks which the private market cannot insure, or cannot insure well (this chapter argues that long-term care is one); and the risks can change over time. Atkinson (1995: 210) points out that

the set of contingencies over which people formed probabilities years ago may have excluded the breakdown of the extended family, or the development of modern medicine, simply because they were inconceivable.

Thus social insurance, in sharp contrast with actuarial insurance, can cover not only risk but also uncertainty.

The rest of this section discusses three approaches to financing long-term care: taxpayer finance; social insurance during working life, that is, *ex ante* social insurance; and social insurance *ex post*, for example a single premium paid out of a person's estate.

Taxpayer finance

Some countries (Germany) finance health care through social insurance, others (the UK) mainly through general taxation, with no explicit contribution. Analogous options exist for long-term care. Germany, as discussed in Rothgang (this issue), uses social insurance. Scandinavia mainly uses tax finance; so does England, though parsimoniously, and Scotland.

It is not surprising that the stress point for this approach is fiscal pressures. The argument against taxpayer finance of long-term care is less one of principle than that of the practical politics of maintaining salience in the competition for public funds. Health care is better placed in this context, since many of its users are articulate and well-connected. It is no accident that social care, not health care, is sometimes described as the 'Cinderella service'.

Social insurance during working life

The approach. This strategy extends existing mandatory social insurance. Workers pay a higher social insurance contribution during working life to finance long-term care. In this approach:

- social insurance covers the costs of (a) meeting clinical need, and (b) providing good-quality 'hotel' care.
- the individual meets the extra costs of hotel care above that provided by the social insurance arrangements – the purpose of social insurance is to finance good-quality care but, given resource constraints, not gourmet food or life in a stately home.

This chapter makes no attempt to set out the detailed workings of this strategy, and so offers no definition of the boundary between 'good-quality' and 'higher-standard' hotel care.[9]

Public pensions take no account of the fact that women on average live longer than men, and the requirement to use unisex life tables has been extended to mandatory private pensions in many countries, including the EU and North America. There are several reasons for adopting this approach for long-term care. First, if insurance is mandatory, there is little or no distortionary effect from charging men and women a premium based on joint probabilities; in particular, adverse selection is not a major problem. Second, there are obvious political difficulties from imposing on women a significantly higher contribution rate than men, all the more since the differential is, and is likely to remain, much larger than for pensions. Finally, the use of unisex tables can be defended as a simple value judgement.

The advantages of this approach are those of social insurance, outlined earlier. First, the system can adjust to changing realities, that is, can address uncertainty. If the incidence of dementia increases sharply the system can accommodate the change, for instance by increasing social insurance contributions. Second, any restrictions on cover have democratic legitimacy, for example legislative change to tighten eligibility rules as a response to medical advances that prolong people's independence.

The German system. Germany has a system of this sort, whereby workers pay an extra 1.95 per cent on their social security contribution.[10] The system pays three different levels of benefit, depending on the extent of the person's incapacity, and offers three types of benefit: in-kind domiciliary care, cash to allow a person to buy his or her own domiciliary care, and residential care. There are additional benefits, for example for adapting a person's house or to cover the costs of respite care.

These arrangements, it can be argued, have the following advantages:

- The system covers the entire population.

- Contributions, at 1.95 per cent of income, are based on ability to pay.
- The system provides help for informal carers through the cash benefit and also by paying the pension contributions of anyone who provides informal care for at least 14 hours a week.
- The contribution mechanism offers some protection against demographic change, in that the additional 1.95 per cent contribution is paid not only by workers but also by pensioners.
- The system widens and deepens the market for care.
- Restrictions on benefit have democratic legitimacy.
- The system is based on an existing administrative mechanism.

For an update of the reform in the German long-term care insurance system see Rothgang (this volume).

Social insurance ex post

It has been proposed (Lloyd 2008) that long-term care could be financed via social insurance, with the premium paid as a lump sum either at age 65 or out of a person's estate. The idea behind this proposal is twofold: as a person gets older, the range of uncertainty about the probability of needing long-term care (p_1 in equation (2)) becomes smaller; and if a person can buy insurance for a single premium payable out of his or her estate, the cost of long-term care does not impinge on his or her living standard during working life or in retirement, but can frequently be taken from housing wealth.

This approach faces a number of questions.

Should membership be voluntary? There is ample evidence from the pensions literature, drawing on lessons from the economics of information (Barr and Diamond 2008: box 4.2) and behavioural economics (2008: box 9.6), that when choices are complex, people make bad choices or no choice at all. Many people realize that they need to save more for their old-age security and intend to so do – but somehow it never happens. In Sweden, workers are required to choose the provider of the private element of their pension, there being over 750 such providers; workers who make no choice are allocated to the default fund; in 2005, some 90 per cent of new workers in Sweden made no choice and were placed in the default fund (Sweden Ministry of Finance 2005: 36).

It would take courage to argue that voluntary choices about long-term care insurance would be any better. The issue is complex, as explained earlier, and people tend to procrastinate.

Compulsion makes politicians nervous, but has significant economic advantages:

- It recognizes the evidence from behavioural economics that people do not always make decisions in their own self-interest.
- It avoids adverse selection, since good risks cannot opt out and bad risks cannot choose to buy inefficiently large amounts of cover.
- A system that is compulsory allows some redistribution; thus it is possible to charge a contribution of x per cent of earnings, respecting ability to pay.

The political problems of compulsion should not be exaggerated. First, contributions for long-term care are smaller than for pensions, since the probability of needing long-term care is lower than that of reaching pensionable age and, where a person needs care, the average duration is less than the average length of time for which a person receives a pension (in the terminology of equation (2) both p_1 and p_2 are smaller for long-term care than for pensions). Second, the pill of compulsion can be sweetened if it is possible to top up the benefits from the compulsory system with privately financed benefits.

An option intermediate between voluntarism and compulsion is to allow self-insurance or only partial insurance for (say) the first two years of needing care; the mandatory social insurance system would pay the costs beyond two years.

Prepayment or post-payment? Should a person pay the single premium at (say) age 65 or be allowed to pay retrospectively out of his/her estate? There are two questions. First, should a person be allowed to *decide* later whether or not to insure? The answer is clear: insurance works only behind the Veil of Ignorance, that is, people have to precommit. Allowing a person to decide later whether to insure creates insoluble problems of adverse selection, since the only people who buy insurance are those who find that they need long-term care – the system degenerates into self-insurance through the insurance equivalent of Gresham's Law.[11]

A different question is whether a person should be allowed to *pay* later. The economic answer is that, so long as the decision to participate has been made earlier, allowing people to pay later is compatible with insurance; what is necessary is a premium whose present value equals the average cost of care.

The political answer, however, is different. Allowing people to pay retrospectively is political dynamite, because many people do not understand the idea of insurance. People may not need long-term care, but when they die the single premium is a claim on their estate. And what if the payment absorbs their entire estate? What about a person who chooses to pay on his/her 65th birthday and dies three weeks later? What about the incentives for a person to give away his or her entire estate?

Conclusion

Earlier discussion suggests powerful analogies with health care: delivery can be public, private or mixed; on finance there is a strong case for relying mainly on public finance. These conclusions are technical rather than ideological.

More specifically, the analysis in this article suggests robust conclusions about the finance of long-term care.

- Self-finance (i.e. financing long-term care out of personal savings or a long-term care savings account) is an inferior solution. Where someone is risk-averse the possibility of pooling risk is welfare-enhancing.
- Actuarial private insurance, for technical reasons – largely connected with information failures in insurance markets – is badly suited to the risks

involved in long-term care, in particular the risk that a person will need such care (p_1 in equation (2)).

- Taxpayer finance is implausible in the English context; it is also implausible elsewhere, given competing fiscal demands connected with population ageing, notably rising spending pressures for pensions and health care, and given global competitive pressures. These long-term trends are all quite separate from the current economic crisis.

- *Ex post* social insurance: a mandatory system in which people pay a single premium at (say) age 65 or out of their estate could work in economic terms, but the political difficulties are likely to be insurmountable. This is all the more the case, since the gain from an *ex post* system, as opposed to an *ex ante* system, is very limited.

- *Ex ante* social insurance: there is a strong case for extending social insurance to provide mandatory cover for long-term care. Social insurance is able to address the major insurance-market problems discussed earlier, is well understood politically, and in administrative terms piggybacks on to existing arrangements. Such a system should be large enough to cover all, or almost all, the costs of a good standard of care, covering both clinical needs and 'hotel' costs. Topping up should be an option, either from private saving or through supplementary private insurance, if that is available on terms that people are prepared to pay. Topping up can be defended both because people have very different tastes, and as a political price for a mandatory system that covers everyone. As with other elements of social insurance, and increasingly with private insurance, the system should be based on unisex probabilities.

Acknowledgements

This chapter draws on Barr (2001: chs 2 and 5). I am grateful to an anonymous referee for helpful comments on an earlier version.

Notes

1. More formally, with risk the probability distribution of outcomes can be estimated with a relatively small variance; with uncertainty, the variance is large.
2. The government can issue indexed bonds to deal with inflation; that, however, is not actuarial insurance, but tax-financed state intervention to assist private insurance.
3. The problem can sometimes be sidestepped in group schemes, where the insurer can impose a pooling solution.
4. Thus p_2 abstracts from the probability of needing care (i.e. p_1); once a person needs care, p_2 addresses the probability distribution of different durations of care.
5. It is well not to get too enthusiastic about tax incentives. Lessons from behavioural economics explain why tax incentives do not have a major effect on pension saving; but such incentives are expensive and can easily be regressive.
6. The relative price effect (in the context of medical care also referred to as excess medical inflation) measures the extent to which the prices of services tend to rise

faster than prices generally. There are two reasons: the price of labour tends to rise faster than the general price level (i.e. real earnings rise); second, services like health care and education have a higher-than-average direct labour content (see Baumol 1996). The argument applies at least as much to care services.

7. For fuller discussion, see, for example, Barr (2001: ch. 4, section 2.2).

8. On retirement as a social construct, see Hannah (1986).

9. In this simple case, co-payments are zero or 100 per cent. It is possible to envisage intermediate options, with different rates of co-payment depending on (a) policy-makers' views about how essential a particular service is, and (b) the extent of the person's dependence. Given potential problems of transparency and hence political sustainability, such a policy is best regarded as a potential future agenda item.

10. Since 2004, a person who has never had any children pays an additional 0.25 per cent.

11. According to Gresham's law, bad money drives out good. If insurers cannot distinguish high- and low-risk buyers, the people who buy insurance will tend to be the bad risks, pushing up insurance premiums and driving out the good risks, who do not find it worth insuring at the higher price.

References

Akerlof, G. A. (1970), The market for 'lemons': qualitative uncertainty and the market mechanism, *Quarterly Journal of Economics*, 84 (August): 488–500 (repr. in N. Barr (ed.) (2001), *Economic Theory and the Welfare State*. Vol. I, *Theory*, Cheltenham: Edward Elgar, pp. 308–20).

Arrow, K. F. (1963), Uncertainty and the welfare economics of medical care, *American Economic Review*, 53: 941–73 (repr. in N. Barr (ed.) (2001), *Economic Theory and the Welfare State*. Vol. I: *Theory*, Cheltenham: Edward Elgar, pp. 275–307).

Atkinson, A. B. (1995), *Incomes and the Welfare State: Essays on Britain and Europe*, Cambridge: Cambridge University Press.

Barr, N. (2001), *The Welfare State as Piggy Bank: Information, Risk, Uncertainty and the Role of the State*, Oxford and New York: Oxford University Press.

Barr, N. and Diamond, P. (2008), *Reforming Pensions: Principles and Policy Choices*, New York and Oxford: Oxford University Press. Available at: www.oxfordscholarship. com/oso/public/content/economicsfinance/9780195311303/toc.html?q= barr|diamond

Baumol, W. (1996), Children of the performing arts, the economics dilemma: the climbing costs of health care and education, *Journal of Cultural Economics*, 20, 3: 183–206.

Burchardt, T. and Hills, J. (1997), *Private Welfare Insurance and Social Security: Pushing the Boundaries*, York: Joseph Rowntree Foundation.

Hannah, L. (1986), *Inventing Retirement*, Cambridge: Cambridge University Press.

Hayek, F. A. (1945), The use of knowledge in society, *American Economic Review*, 35: 519–30.

Lloyd, J. (2008), *Funding Long-term Care: The Building Blocks of Reform*, London: International Longevity Centre–UK. Available at: www.ilcuk.org.uk.

Lucas, R. E. (1987), *Models of Business Cycles*, Oxford: Basil Blackwell.

Nuttall, S., Blackwood, R., Bussell, B., Cliff, J., Conrall, M., Cowley, A., Gatenby, P. and Webber, J. (1995), Financing long-term care in Great Britain, *Journal of the Institute of Actuaries*, 121, 1: 1–68.

Pauly, M. V. (1990), The rational non-purchase of long-term care insurance, *Journal of Political Economy*, 98, 1: 153–68.

Rawls, J. (1972), *A Theory of Justice*, Oxford: Oxford University Press.

Sloan, F. A. and Norton, E. C. (1997), Adverse selection bequests, crowding out, and private demand for insurance: evidence from the long-term care insurance market, *Journal of Risk and Uncertainty*, 15, 3: 201–19.

Sweden Ministry of Finance (2005), Difficult waters: premium pension savings on course (Premium Pension Committee, SOU 2005:87), Stockholm. Available at: www.sweden.gov.se/sb/d/574/a/52265;jsessionid=alkgAkqIj71g.

UK Royal Commission on Long Term Care (1999), *With Respect to Old Age: A Report by the Royal Commission on Long Term Care*, Cm 4192-I, London: Stationery Office.

2

The Long Road to Universalism? Recent Developments in the Financing of Long-term Care in England

Adelina Comas-Herrera, Raphael Wittenberg and Linda Pickard

Introduction

The financing of long-term care (LTC) has been among the most debated social policy issues in England for the last decade (Royal Commission on Long Term Care 1999; Brooks *et al.* 2002; JRF 2006; Wanless *et al.* 2006). Underlying the debate are concerns both about the future affordability of LTC and about the fairness of the current funding system. The key issue in the financing debate is how far people should fund their own care and how far they should be publicly funded, in particular whether public funds for LTC should benefit only those who cannot afford to pay for themselves (a residual model) or whether free LTC should be a universal entitlement. The debate started from before the establishment of the Royal Commission on Long Term Care (1999) and has continued, more or less unabated, since then. One reason why the debate has been so intense is because, for the last seven years, there have been different systems of LTC in different parts of the United Kingdom. LTC is a devolved responsibility to the nations of the United Kingdom, and in Scotland the central recommendation of the Royal Commission on Long Term Care was adopted and free personal care was introduced in 2002. In the rest of the UK, however, free personal care has not, at the time of writing, been introduced. The debate over LTC in England has intensified since the publication of the Wanless social care review, which argued in favour of a 'partnership' model of funding personal care, whereby the costs of care would be shared partly by the state and partly by the individual (Wanless *et al.* 2006). The debate over long-term care has come to a head in England in recent months with the government's publication of a Green Paper, *Shaping the Future of Care Together*, which is currently consulting on potentially radical changes (HM Government 2009), and with the government's announcement of a policy of free personal care in their own homes for people with the highest needs to be introduced in autumn 2010 (*Community Care* 2009b).

The first part of this chapter examines key issues relating to the current LTC system in England, exploring both the problems identified in the Green

Paper and other issues identified in the wider social policy literature. The second part discusses recent reviews and reports recommending reform of the financing system, including the proposals contained in the Green Paper. The chapter aims to present a broad overview of the current organizational structures in England, to discuss the key suggested reforms and to put them in an international context. Since responsibility for health and social care in the United Kingdom is, as already implied, devolved to the administrations for each country, this chapter concentrates on England, but references are also made to the systems in Scotland, Wales and Northern Ireland.

The Current System

In international comparisons the English long-term care system has been characterized as a 'safety-net' (Fernández *et al.* 2009) or 'residual' (Brodsky *et al.* 2003) system that only supports those with very severe needs who are unable to meet the costs of their care. It is also a system that has evolved incrementally from earlier systems of welfare for the poor by developing specific services to meet the LTC needs of older people and a limited relaxation of the means tests (Ikegami and Campbell 2002). Partly as a result of its origins, it is a complex system that most people do not understand. A recent review of eligibility criteria for social care in England by the former Commission for Social Care Inspection (CSCI) concluded that there is 'a lack of clarity and transparency in practice, particularly relating to the complexity of the framework, so neither professionals nor people using services are confident of their understanding' (CSCI 2008: 4).

Long-term care in the UK is usually taken to mean help with domestic tasks, such as shopping and preparing meals, assistance with personal care tasks, such as dressing and bathing, and nursing care. There is a mixed economy of provision of care. The system relies heavily on informal or unpaid care provided by family, friends or neighbours (Pickard *et al.* 2000, 2007). Formal services are provided by a range of agencies including local authority social services, community health services and independent (for- and non-profit) sector residential care homes, nursing homes, home-care and day-care services. There is also a mixed economy of finance. Services are financed by the National Health Service, local authorities, charities and older people themselves. While health-care services are free at the point of use, social care is means-tested. There is a non-means-tested disability benefit for older people with personal care needs and a benefit for carers.

Access to publicly funded services is mainly through an assessment of care needs coordinated by the local authority social services department. Assessment and care management aim to determine eligibility for publicly funded care and develop a care package to meet assessed needs. There has been an emphasis on targeting services to people with greater disabilities. A care manager may be involved in coordinating the assessment and organization of care and may have a devolved budget with which to purchase services. People assessed as eligible for a package of care can instead opt for a direct payment that they can use to buy equipment or services themselves. In 2006/7, some 460,000 older people not already in receipt of services had a completed assessment of their needs (Department of Health 2008). Most of the referrals (for people of all ages) were self-referrals (29 per cent), followed by secondary health services (23 per cent), from family, friends or neighbours (14 per cent) and from primary or community health (13 per cent). After first contact, 62 per cent of older people had their completed assessment within two weeks and 94 per cent within three months (Department of Health 2008).

Following an assessment, a person may be provided with a new service, may not be offered a service, may themselves decline any service, or may have some other outcome. Some may be referred on to NHS or housing agencies or to voluntary sector services. In 2006/7, most older people assessed as eligible (79 per cent) received all their services within two weeks after the assessment (Department of Health 2008).

Eligibility criteria for publicly funded social care, arrangements for assessments and budgets are determined locally and there is great variability between local authorities. In 2002 the Department of Health published a national framework for eligibility criteria, *Fair Access to Care Services*, to address inconsistencies across the country (Department of Health 2002). The aim of the framework was to ensure that people with similar needs would be able to achieve similar outcomes. It did not require individuals with similar needs to be given similar services. The framework provided four severity bands (low, moderate, substantial and critical) to which individuals are allocated. Councils can choose where to set their eligibility criteria within those bands.

The eligibility criteria have tightened considerably over recent years, partly as a result of budgetary constraints. Most councils only consider eligible those in the substantial and critical bands and some only those in the critical band. The report by the former CSCI, mentioned earlier, found that, despite the implementation of the eligibility framework, there are still wide variations between councils (CSCI 2008). Another report by the Audit Commission (2008) on the effects of the *Fair Access to Care Services* system on expenditure and service provision found that there were wide variations in spending on care for older people, according to how restrictive the use of thresholds was. There are concerns that the needs of people in the more moderate bands are not being met and that opportunities for prevention are being missed, leading to worse outcomes for care users and higher costs to the system (Wanless *et al.* 2006; CSCI 2008; HM Government 2009). In 2007 the government published a ministerial concordat, *Putting People First*, which aims at changing the emphasis of the system towards early intervention and prevention (HM Government 2007). Consultations are currently under way to find a means of ensuring that the Fair Access to Care Services system fully supports this change in direction (Department of Health 2009: 10).

Eligibility for publicly funded care and support takes into account the availability of informal care, so that older people with similar levels of disability do not receive the same amounts of formal service support. Services in England are primarily directed at disabled older people who do not receive informal care, particularly those who live alone (Arber *et al.* 1988; McNamee *et al.* 1999; Evandrou 2005). Since the majority of disabled older people in England either live with others and/or receive informal care (see table 1), eligibility criteria restricting formal service support primarily to those living alone or those without informal care are an important reason why many disabled older people are currently not considered eligible for publicly funded support (see table 2). As a consequence, unlike a number of other LTC systems in Western Europe, the system in England is not 'carer-blind' (Pickard 2001; Fernández *et al.* 2009). The fact that eligibility criteria take into account the availability of informal care in England has been a source of criticism of the LTC system in this country (Royal Commission on Long Term Care 1999; Himmelweit and Land 2008; Glendinning and Bell 2008).

Those people who have been assessed as eligible for social care services are then subject to a means test to establish whether their services will be funded wholly or partly by the local authority. There is a national charging regime for residential and nursing home care in England, which takes into account the income and assets (in most cases including any housing wealth) of residents. Those with assets over an upper limit, currently set at £23,000, are not eligible for local authority support. Those with assets below this level are required to contribute most of their income towards the costs of their care. The NHS makes a non-means-tested contribution for nursing costs in care homes.

Local authorities have discretion over whether and how they charge for home care services, although there are national guidelines (Department of Health 2003) which set out common principles to which local authorities must adhere in determining how much to charge users. In particular they must disregard a sum of income equivalent to at least 25 per cent above the level of social security income maintenance benefits.

Table 1

People with a functional disability in private households aged 65 and over, by marital status, household type and receipt of informal care, England, 2006 (estimated numbers in thousands and column percentages)

Marital status, household type and receipt of informal care	Numbers	Column (%)
Single, living alone, no informal care	205,000	10
Single, living alone, receives informal care	670,000	32
Single, living with child, receives informal care	160,000	8
Single, living with others, receives informal care	55,000	3
Couple, no informal care	75,000	4
Couple, receives informal care from spouse	695,000	34
Couple, receives informal care from child	100,000	5
Couple, living with others, receives informal care	110,000	5
All disabled in households	*2,068,000*	*100*

Notes: Numbers are rounded to nearest 5,000. 'People with a functional disability' are defined as those having difficulties with instrumental or basic Activities of Daily Living, or needing help with one Activity of Daily Living. 'Single' refers to widowed, divorced, separated and never married people who are not cohabiting; 'couple' refers to those living in legal or *de facto* partnerships.
Source: PSSRU model estimates, based on data from the 2001/2 GHS and 2006 official population data.

Table 2

Estimated number of older people receiving services in a given day by service type and age, England, 2006–7

	Number of users	% of older population
Day care	93,000	1.15
Meals	229,000	2.83
Local authority arr. home care	293,000	3.62
Respite care	24,000	0.30
Private home care	150,000[1]	
Community nursing	445,000[1]	5.50
Direct payments	18,000[2]	0.22
Professional support	101,000	1.25
Equipment and adaptation	136,000	1.68
Independent sector residential care	179,000	2.21
Local authority residential care	22,000	0.27
Nursing care homes	127,000	1.57
Long-stay hospital	9,000	0.11
All in institutions	*337,000*	*4.17*

[1]Estimates from the PSSRU LTC model, based on levels of service receipt report in the 2001/2 General Household Survey. Note that the definition of private help used here only includes those who needed help with one or more ADLs.
[2]27,000 in 2007–8.
Source: Department of Health (2008a: 6). There is overlap between home-based services.

Services are provided by local authority and independent providers. In the last 10 years there has been a fast increase in the amount of care provided by private providers (Philpott 2008; NHS Information Centre 2009). Prices are negotiated between the local authorities and the providers, except in the case of clients with direct payments, who negotiate directly with the providers. People can also buy services directly from private providers, without any mediation from the public sector. There are concerns that, where the fees paid by local authorities are low, providers set higher prices for private payers, which means that, effectively, private payers are subsidizing local authority-funded services (Netten *et al.* 2003).

Around 325,000 older people, some 4 per cent of the older population of England, are residents in care homes. These comprise 192,000 local authority-funded residents, an estimated 105,000 privately funded residents and an estimated 29,000 NHS-funded residents. Around 650,000 older people receive local authority-funded community-based services, including some 300,000 receiving home care. An estimated 150,000 severely disabled older people (unable to conduct personal care tasks without help) purchase home care privately, with substantially larger numbers of less disabled older people purchasing private help. Further details are at table 2.

Services are heavily concentrated on the oldest old. Those over age 85 are more likely to receive all formal services than the 'younger' old, and this is

Table 3

Key characteristics of recipients of domiciliary and residential care, compared to the general population of older people, Great Britain, 2002

	All older people (aged 65 and over) (%)	Recipients of community services* (%)	Recipients of residential care (%)
Aged 85 and over	12	26	52
Female	58	66	76
Living alone**	38	65	68
Owner-occupier**	68	73	43

*Covering home care and private domestic help services.
**For people in care homes, household type and housing tenure are prior to admission.
Source: PSSRU model estimates, using ONS population estimates and analyses of 2001/2 GHS, Department of Health and PSSRU residential care survey data.

particularly true of residential care (table 3). Recipients of residential care are also more likely to have lived alone prior to admission to care and are less likely to have owned their own homes (Hancock et al. 2002).

In the context of a general national policy of extending individual consumer choice in the public sector (6, 2003), and in line with developments in other countries (Lundsgaard 2005; Pavolini and Ranci 2008), reforms are under way to give people entitled to publicly funded social care services choice and control over their care. These reforms started with the introduction of a form of cash payments called direct payments in 1997 for adult disabled people and the extension to older people in 2000. Direct payments are available to people who have been assessed as needing services and are eligible for publicly funded support. The level of a direct payment is calculated according to the amount of personal support needed by the individual and costed with reference to the costs of equivalent services in kind. They are commonly used by recipients to employ a personal assistant or helper to provide the support they need. The employment of close relatives living in the same household is not allowed, except in exceptional circumstances. The purchase of services from the local authority is not allowed either. The take-up of direct payments, specially among older people, has been low. Numerous barriers have been identified, including the restrictions on the use of the payments, the administrative burden of becoming an employer, lack of effective support schemes for users and reluctance of local authorities to promote direct payments (Davey et al. 2007).

In 2007 the government published a ministerial concordat called *Putting People First*, which sets out reforms to personalize social care. The document states that 'the time has now come to build on best practice and replace paternalistic, reactive care of variable quality with a mainstream system focussed on prevention, early intervention, enablement, and high quality personally tailored services. In the future, we want people to have maximum choice, control and power over the support services they receive' (HM Government 2007: 2). A fundamental component of the reform is personal budgets: an individual allocation of funding to enable individuals to make choices about how best to meet their needs, including their broader health and well-being. A person will be able to take all or part of their personal budget as a direct payment, to pay for their own support either by employing individuals themselves or by purchasing support through an agency. Others may wish, once they have decided on their preferred care package, to have the council continue to pay for this directly. It is possible to have a combination of both approaches. The *Putting People First* reforms aim at reducing the barriers to take-up that direct payments have encountered. Personal budgets present much lower demands to the individuals in terms of employing and managing people (Samuel 2009). They are also accompanied by targets and a substantial 'Social Care Reform Grant' to local authorities to help them redesign and reshape their services (Department of Health 2009).

There has also been a large-scale pilot of another system of cash payment called individual budget (IB). IBs were piloted in 13 local authorities as a new system of cash payments that would bring together, for any individual, the resources from a number of different services or funding streams that they are entitled to. These resources include local authority funding for social care, community equipment and housing adaptations and other disability-related benefits (but not Attendance Allowance or NHS funding). An individual budget would pool these resources for any one person and the total amount would be made transparent to the individual. The individual budget could be used to secure a flexible range of goods and services, from a wider variety of providers than is possible with direct payments. For example, the IB could be used to pay informal carers living in the same household, or to purchase goods or services from local authorities. A national evaluation found that IB resources were typically used to pay for personal care, domestic help and social, leisure and educational activities. Most people chose to purchase conventional forms of support. The evaluation found that overall, holding an IB was associated with better social care outcomes, but older people reported lower psychological well-being with IBs, perhaps because they felt the processes of planning and managing their own support were burdens (Glendinning *et al.* 2008). The government has only called for the roll-out of personal budgets, not individual budgets.

Total expenditure on long-term care services for older people in England has been estimated, using the PSSRU macrosimulation model, to be £17.75 billion in 2006 (or 1.49 per cent of Gross Domestic Product [GDP]). Of this, 20.6 per cent was funded by local authorities (personal social services), and 39.7 per cent by individuals or their families (of which 10 per cent were user charges and 29.7 per cent were direct private expenditures). This figure does not include the contribution of informal carers, or contributions by charities.

Another important component of the care system is social security disability benefits. Attendance Allowance, and Disability Living Allowance for those who started to receive disability benefits from before the age of 65, are the main disability benefits for older people with disabilities. In 2006/7 these benefits paid out £4.2 billion. Attendance allowance is paid at two rates, depending on whether the older person needs assistance during the day (2006/7, £43.15 a week) and/or night (£64.50), and is not means-tested. In 2006, some 1.59 million people were receiving Attendance Allowance in England. Eligibility for Attendance Allowance is governed by the need for help or supervision, but the claimant does not actually have to be in receipt of such support. It is a compensation for disability rather than a payment to cover the costs of services. Analysis of data from the English Longitudinal Study of Ageing (ELSA) showed that only a minority (27 per cent) of Attendance Allowance claimants used either state-funded or privately funded social care. Some 29 per cent were receiving neither formal nor informal care (Wanless et al. 2006: 94).

The long-term care system in the UK has been characterized as one in which there is 'extensive financial support for informal care' (Lundsgaard 2005). Financial support for informal care in this country takes the form of Carers' Allowance, a non-means-tested benefit paid to people providing long hours of informal care. The allowance, which amounts to £53.10 a week, is paid to informal carers who provide at least 35 hours informal care per week, earn less than £95 per week, are not in full-time education and look after someone who receives qualifying disability benefits (such as Attendance Allowance). Carers' Allowance is based on a social security model of payments for care (Glendinning and McLaughlin 1993) and is regarded by the Department for Work and Pensions as a compensation for loss of earnings, not as a wage for caring. There were approximately 365,000 recipients of Carers' Allowance in England in 2005, and UK expenditure on the allowance was approximately £1.3 billion in 2007/8 (NAO 2009). Carers' Allowance (and its predecessor, Invalid Care Allowance) has long been the subject of criticism in this country, primarily because of its low level and its poor coverage of heavily committed carers (Pickard 1999; NAO 2009).

In addition to social security support, there are national policies intended to provide support for informal carers in England. Indeed, there has been an increasing emphasis in government policy over the last two decades on providing support for informal carers (Pickard 2001; Beesley 2006). Current policies are embodied in a new national strategy for carers entitled *Carers at the Heart of 21st-Century Families and Communities* (HM Government 2008). The policy emphasis is primarily on provision of 'carer-support services' to enable informal carers to continue providing care. Since the mid-1990s, people providing substantial and regular care in England have had the right to a local authority assessment of their needs for services and, since 2001, they have been entitled to receive services in their own right (Beesley 2006). However, only a minority of 'heavy duty' carers receive assessments and only around one in ten receives carer-support services (*ibid.*).

Financing Long-term Care: Key Suggested Reforms

The government considered the issue of long-term care funding sufficiently important and complex to warrant the first Royal Commission for many years. The purpose of the Royal Commission on Long Term Care was to review the financing of LTC and to make recommendations about future financing. Its key recommendation, as indicated at the beginning of this chapter, was that there should be 'free' personal and nursing care, that is, the nursing and personal care components of the fees of care homes and home-based personal care should be met by the state, without a means test, and financed out of general taxation (Royal Commission on Long Term Care 1999). Means-testing would remain for the accommodation and ordinary living costs ('hotel' costs) covered by residential fees and for help with domestic tasks. The report of the Royal Commission also recommended that 'the Government ensure services become increasingly "carer blind"' (Royal Commission on Long Term Care 1999: 90).

The government accepted some of the Royal Commission's recommendations but only removed the means test for nursing care in nursing homes (Secretary of State for Health 2000). Similar decisions were adopted by the National Assembly for Wales and the Northern Ireland Assembly. However, as indicated earlier, the Scottish Executive decided that it would make personal care for older people free of charge as well (Care Development Group 2001).

These decisions did not bring an end to the debate about how best to fund LTC. Pressure to make personal care free of charge throughout the UK remained. A left-leaning think tank, the Institute for Public Policy Research (IPPR), for example, advocated that personal care should be made free to all (Brooks *et al.* 2002). The Joseph Rowntree Foundation (JRF) conducted a major three-year programme on paying for LTC in the UK and argued strongly for better funding arrangements, describing the policy of free personal care in Scotland as 'promising', 'popular' and 'perceived as fair' (JRF 2006: 2). The JRF, though stressing the need for fundamental reform of the system, has also suggested a number of ways in which the present system could be improved without incurring excessive costs (Hirsch 2005; JRF 2006).

The King's Fund set up in 2005 a review of care for older people, under the leadership of Sir Derek Wanless, to determine how much should be spent on social care for older people in England over the coming 20 years. The report of the review, *Securing Good Care for Older People*, was published in 2006 (Wanless *et al.* 2006). As indicated earlier, the Wanless review favoured a partnership arrangement 'characterised by combining a publicly funded entitlement to a guaranteed level of care, with a variable component made up of contributions from individuals matched at a given rate by contributions from the state' (2006: 278). Wanless proposed that the publicly funded entitlement should be two-thirds of the benchmark level of care. Users could choose whether they wanted the remaining third, with the costs being met half by the user and half by the state. The benchmark level of care is the level that is cost-effective given a cost-effectiveness threshold of £20,000 per ADLAY (that is, the gain for one year of life of having core activities of daily living [ADL] needs improved from being entirely unmet to being fully met). A partnership arrangement on these lines would require an increase in public expenditure of some £3.5 billion.

The Wanless report advocates a partnership model because it believes that, on balance, it compares favourably to free personal care or a means-tested system.

27

- the Wanless report argues that the partnership model is efficient. It suggests that it produces the highest ratio of outcomes (ADLAYs) to costs of the three funding systems (Wanless *et al.* 2006: 270);
- it has strengths and weaknesses in regard to equity and fairness: 'for the guaranteed element, support is based entirely on need and not ability to pay, but the converse is largely the case for the matched element' (2006: 269);
- it scores well on choice, as individuals will be able to choose the level of care they receive above the guaranteed level, albeit subject to co-payment;
- it scores as well as free personal care on dignity, as no means-testing would be required within the care system;
- it is not as strong as a means-tested system on economic sustainability, but if necessary 'the guaranteed entitlement can be scaled back to reduce costs . . . or the matching contribution can be reduced' (2006: 271), and more options for dealing with sustainability could be added;
- it is not as strong as free personal care in terms of introducing a 'carer-blind' approach, since the partnership model is not 'carer-blind', whereas free personal care is described as partially so in the Wanless review (2006: 246).

The Wanless review prompted renewed interest in the financing of long-term care. In February 2008 the International Longevity Centre–UK set out a proposal for funding older people's LTC based around a social insurance fund for the retirement stage, into which individuals would make contributions as a lump-sum, through regular instalments or as a charge on their estate (Lloyd 2008). In this volume, Nicholas Barr proposes the extension of social insurance to provide mandatory cover for LTC, with the possibility of topping up either from private savings or through supplementary private insurance (see Barr, this volume).

During 2008, the government ran a six-month engagement process on the care and support system in England. This involved seeking the views of the public, service users and staff. It was followed in July 2009 by the publication of the Green Paper (HM Government 2009), which sets out the government's proposals for ways to reform the care and support system for adults in England.

The Green Paper lists a number of problems with the current LTC system, which the proposed reforms are intended to address (2009: 8). A key problem is that many older and disabled people in England do not get any help from the state towards paying for their care and support, partly because publicly funded social care is means-tested (*ibid.*). The means test for long-stay residential care includes the value of the older or disabled person's house, which means that many older people in need of residential care have to 'sell their homes to pay for care and support' (*ibid.*). In addition, state-funded care and support is often provided only when people have already developed high levels of need, therefore allowing preventative opportunities to be missed (*ibid.*). Moreover, people with the same needs receive different levels of care depending on where they live; the different parts of the care and support system do not work together; the care system as a whole is confusing and the system is not tailored to people's needs (*ibid.*). Problems associated with the current system are expected to be exacerbated in the coming years by the growing numbers of older people, with the Green Paper estimating that 1.7 million more adults will need care and support by 2026 (2009: 9).

The Green Paper states the government intention to build the first National Care Service in England. The vision is 'for a system that is fair, simple and affordable for everyone, underpinned by national rights and entitlements but personalised to individual needs' (2009: 9). The proposals extend beyond the financing system, to cover:

- prevention services, encompassing free support to stay well and as independent as possible;
- national assessment, which will give people the right to have their care needs assessed in the same way wherever they live in England and to have the same proportion of their care and support costs met;
- a joined-up service, such that people will need to have only one assessment of their care needs to gain access to a range of care and support services which will work together smoothly;
- information and advice to help people find their way around the care and support system;
- personalized care and support, with care and support designed around individual needs;
- fair funding, where everyone who qualifies for care and support from the state will get help meeting the cost of care and support needs.

The Green Paper discusses five possible funding options:

- pay for yourself, under which there would be no support from the state;
- partnership, where everyone who qualified for care and support would be entitled to have a set proportion of their basic care and support costs met by the state, with that proportion inversely related to the person's resources;
- insurance, which would comprise the partnership system plus insurance for those wanting to purchase it;
- comprehensive, where everyone over retirement age who had the resources to do so would be required to pay into a state insurance scheme;
- tax-funded system, which would provide free care funded from increased general taxation.

The Green Paper rules out the first and last of these options and consults on the other three. Because the first option is ruled out, the Green Paper is in essence proposing that 'everyone who has high levels of care and support need gets *some* of their care and support paid for by the state' (HM Government 2009: 19, emphasis added). In this sense, the underlying model advocated in the Green Paper is the partnership approach. As the Green Paper puts it: 'We think that the Partnership option should be the foundation of the new system' (*ibid.*). The questions then are whether, how far and by what financing mechanism the remaining costs are met (*ibid.*).

Initial responses to the Green Paper suggest that there is likely to be general approval for a National Care Service, but that consultation around the Green Paper is also likely to raise a number of issues for debate (*Community Care* 2009a; *Health Service Journal* 2009; Age Concern/Help the Aged 2009; Scope 2009). One area is likely to be the proportion of care and support needs to be met by the state in either a partnership- or insurance-based option. The Green Paper suggests that the state might meet, for example, a quarter to a third of basic care and support costs (HM Government 2009: 17). This falls considerably short of the two-thirds of the 'benchmark level of care' that Wanless suggested should be met by the state (Wanless *et al.* 2006). Another area of contention is likely to be the Green Paper's suggestion that Attendance Allowance could be integrated into the care and support system (HM Government 2009: 15), a suggestion to which a number of 'stakeholder' organizations have already indicated their opposition (Scope 2009; Age Concern/Help the Aged 2009). A third area of potential concern is likely to be the ruling out of taxation as a means of funding the proposed National Care Service and the confinement of the funding options to contributions from older people alone. The leading organization representing older people in England has argued instead that 'costs must be shared fairly across the generations' (Age Concern/Help the Aged 2009). Funding through social insurance paid during people's working lives, '*ex-ante* social insurance', would, however, share costs across the generations without raising taxation (see Barr, this volume). Finally, the treatment of informal care in the Green Paper may also lead to debate. Although there is little reference to policy for carers in the Green Paper, its proposals are likely to have consequences for informal care. Because the foundation of the proposals in the Green Paper is a partnership approach (HM Government 2009: 19), and because a partnership approach is not 'carer-blind' (Wanless *et al.* 2006: 246), not all the options proposed in the Green Paper would necessarily address concerns, recently expressed, about the dependence of the care and support system on the availability of informal care (Himmelweit and Land 2008; Glendinning and Bell 2008).

At the time of writing, the government has just announced a new policy of free personal care in their own homes for those with the highest needs, to be introduced in the autumn of 2010 (*Community Care* 2009b). According to the information available to the authors at the time of writing, this policy is separate from the proposals contained in the Green Paper and would apply to older people living in private households with critical care needs (*ibid.*). The proposals have been widely welcomed by organizations representing older people and social policy analysts, although some organizations have urged caution until the 'substance behind the sound bite' has been analysed (BBC 2009).

Conclusions

The current UK long-term care system is to a considerable extent many local systems. Health and social care are a devolved function, which means that the responsibility for health and social policy is devolved to the administrations for England, Scotland, Wales and Northern Ireland. Devolution has led to some policy divergence, and key differences have arisen in the funding of social care: in particular, while Scotland has introduced free personal and nursing care, the other countries have introduced only free nursing care.

Responsibility for assessing local needs and commissioning health and social services rests with primary care trusts (PCTs) and local authorities respectively in England, and with their equivalents in the other countries. For social care, local authorities are responsible for assessing population needs, commissioning services, setting local eligibility criteria and assessing individuals against those criteria. While there is a national system for mean-testing and charging for residential care, local authorities determine locally the system for charging and means-testing for home care.

The UK system is marked by a mixed economy of supply. The system relies heavily on informal care provided mainly by close relatives. There is a wide range of providers of formal care in the public, voluntary (not-for-profit) and private (for-profit) sectors. Direct payments, which are cash alternatives to services, are now available to enable people to employ their own carers or to use for a wide range of purposes.

The system is also marked by a mixed economy of finance. Health care, including nursing care in all settings, is free at the point of use, and is funded mainly from general taxation. Most social care (except for personal care for older people in Scotland) is means-tested and is funded by a combination of central taxation, local taxation and user charges. Disability benefits, by contrast, are not means-tested and are funded from general taxation. This means that the system is complex and not easily understood.

It is against this background that the government's Green Paper is currently consulting on a wide range of issues. These comprise not only options for the financing system but also the nature of the new National Care Service, such as the balance between national and local responsibilities and the development of joined-up services. Evidence from elsewhere in this issue suggests that reductions in local fragmentation are, under certain conditions, achievable goals of LTC policy (see Costa-Font, and Trydegård and Thorslund, this volume). Moreover, there is no doubt that the government in England has taken an important step forward in acknowledging the problems in the current LTC system and the need for change. The Green Paper includes options that could address many of the problems with the current system, identified both by the government and more widely. However, the areas of contention are still likely to concern the balance between the individual and the state.

A clear message from the Green Paper is the will to create a new National Care Service, as opposed to many diverse local services, with a national entitlement to some public support to all those who are assessed as needing it. If implemented, the proposals included in the Green Paper would, at minimum, introduce a 'quasi-universal' system, in which some level of assistance is provided to all those with eligible social care needs. Such systems have recently been introduced elsewhere in Europe, such as in France (see Le Bihan and Martin, this volume). 'Quasi-universalism' does not, however, seem to have reduced the pressure for further reform and for the introduction of a universal LTC system (see Le Bihan and Martin, this volume).

With consultation on the Green Paper having closed in November 2009, a White Paper with formal proposals is expected to follow in 2010 with plans for the introduction in England of free personal care at home for people with the highest needs. This promises to be a very interesting time for long-term care in the UK.

References

Age Concern and Help the Aged (2009), Green Paper Sets Out Reform Challenge. Available at: ageconcern.org.uk/AgeConcern/release-care-green-paper-140709.asp, dated 14 July 2009 (accessed 4 September 2009).

Arber, S., Gilbert, G. N. and Evandrou, M. (1988), Gender, household composition and receipt of domiciliary services by elderly disabled people, *Journal of Social Policy*, 17: 153–75.

Audit Commission (2008), The Effect of Fair Access to Care Services Bands on Expenditure and Service Provision. Available at: www.cqc.org.uk/_db/_documents/Tracked%20Audit%20Commission%20report%20on%20FACS%20 13%20August_typeset.pdf.

BBC (2009), 'Free personal care' for elderly (29 September). Available at: http://news.bbc.co.uk/1/hi/health/8281168.stm.

Beesley, L. (2006), *Informal Care in England*, London: King's Fund.

Brodsky, J., Habib, J., Hirschfeld, M., Siegel, B. and Rockoff, Y. (2003), Choosing overall LTC strategies: a conceptual framework for policy development. In WHO, *Key Policy Issues in Long-Term Care*, Geneva: World Health Organization, pp. 245–70.

Brooks, R., Regan, S. and Robinson, P. (2002), *A New Contract for Retirement*, London: Institute for Public Policy Research.

Care Development Group (2001), *Fair Care for Older People*, Edinburgh: Stationery Office.

Commission for Social Care Inspection (CSCI) (2008), *Cutting the Cake Fairly: CSCI Review of Eligibility Criteria for Social Care*, London: CSCI.

Community Care (2009a), Public funding will not increase, DH confirms, *Community Care* (14 July). Available at: www.communitycare.co.uk/Articles/2009/07/14/112101/ adult-green-paper-government-outlines-national-care-service.htm.

Community Care (2009b), Gordon Brown makes free personal care pledge, *Community Care* (29 September). Available at: www.communitycare.co.uk/Articles/2009/ 09/29/112722/gordon-brown-makes-free-personal-care-pledge.htm.

Davey, V., Snell, T., Fernández, J.-L., Knapp, M., Tobin, R., Jolly, D., Perkins, M., Kendall, J., Pearson, C., Vick, N., Swift, P., Mercer, G. and Priestley, M. (2007), *Schemes Providing Support to People Using Direct Payments: A UK Survey*, London: Personal Social Services Research Unit.

Department of Health (2002), *Fair Access to Care Services: Guidance on Eligibility Criteria for Adult Social Care*, London: DH.

Department of Health (2003), Fairer Charging Policies for Home Care and other Non-residential Social Services: Guidance for Councils with Social Care Responsibilities. Available at: www.dh.gov.uk/prod_consum_dh/groups/dh_ digitalassets/@dh/@en/documents/digitalasset/dh_4117931.pdf (accessed 10 September 2009).

Department of Health (2008), *Community Care Statistics 2007–08: Referrals, Assessments and Packages of Care for Adults, England: National Summary*, London: Health and Social Care Information Centre.

Department of Health (2009), *Transforming Adult Social Care* (Local Authority Circular), London: Department of Health. Available at: www.dh.gov.uk/en/Publications andstatistics/Lettersandcirculars/LocalAuthorityCirculars/DH_095719 (accessed 11 September 2009).

Evandrou, M. (2005), Health and social care. In Office for National Statistics (ed.), *Focus on Older People*, London: Stationery Office, pp. 51–65.

Fernández, J.-L., Forder, J., Truckeschitz, B., Rokosova, M. and McDaid, D. (2009), *How Can European States Design Efficient, Equitable and Sustainable Funding Systems for Long-term Care for Older People?* Policy Brief 11, Copenhagen: World Health Organization Europe.

Glendinning, C. and Bell, D. (2008), *Rethinking Social Care and Support: What Can England Learn from Other Countries?* York: Joseph Rowntree Foundation.

Glendinning, C. and McLaughlin, E. (1993), *Paying for Care: Lessons from Europe*, London: HMSO.

Glendinning, C., Challis, D., Fernández, J.-L., Jacobs, S., Knapp, M., Manthorpe, J., Moran, N., Netten, A., Stevens, M. and Wilberforce, M. (2008), *Evaluation of the Individual Budgets Pilot Programme Final Report*, Individual Budgets Evaluation Network. Available from: www.pssru.ac.uk/pdf/IBSEN.pdf.

Hancock, R., Arthur, A., Jagger, C. and Matthews, R. (2002), The effects of older people's economic resources on care home entry under the UK long-term care financing system, *Journals of Gerontology: Social Sciences*, 57B, 5: S285–S293.

Health Service Journal (2009), 'National care service' could pit councils against NHS, *Health Service Journal* (15 July 2009). Available at: www.hsj.co.uk/primary-care/national-care-service-could-pit-councils-against-nhs/5004026.article.

Himmelweit, S. and Land, H. (2008), *Reducing Gender Inequalities to Create a Sustainable Care System*, York: Joseph Rowntree Foundation.

Hirsch, D. (2005), *Facing the Cost of Long-Term Care: Towards a Sustainable Funding System*, York: Joseph Rowntree Foundation.

HM Government (2007), *Putting People First: A Shared Vision and Commitment to the Transformation of Adult Social Care*, London: HMG.

HM Government (2008), *Carers at the Heart of 21st-Century Families and Communities: 'A Caring System on your Side. A Life of your Own'*. London: HMG.

HM Government (2009), *Shaping the Future of Care Together*, London: HMG.

Ikegami, N. and Campbell, J. C. (2002), Choices, policy logics and problems in the design of long-term care systems, *Social Policy & Administration*, 36, 7: 719–34.

Joseph Rowntree Foundation (JRF) (2006), *Paying for Long-Term Care*, York: JRF.

Lloyd, J. (2008), *A National Care Fund for Long-Term Care*, London: International Longevity Centre–UK.

Lundsgaard, J. (2005), *Consumer Direction and Choice in Long-Term Care for Older Persons, Including Payments for Informal Care: How Can it Help Improve Care Outcomes, Employment and Fiscal Sustainability*, OECD Health Working Papers no. 20, DELSA/HEA/WD/HWP(2005)1.

McNamee, P., Gregson, B. A., Buck, D., Bamford, C. H., Bond, J. and Wright, K. (1999), Costs of formal care for frail older people in England: the resource implications study of the MRC cognitive function and ageing study (RIS MRC CFAS), *Social Science and Medicine*, 48: 331–41.

NAO (National Audit Office) (2009), *Department for Work and Pensions: Supporting Carers to Care*, London: Stationery Office.

Netten, A., Darton, R. and Williams, J. (2003), Nursing home closures: effects on capacity and reasons for closure, *Age and Ageing*, 32: 332–7.

NHS Information Centre (2009), *Community Care Statistics 2008: Home Care Services for Adults, England*, Health and Social Care Information Centre. Available at: www.ic. nhs.uk/webfiles/publications/Home%20Care%20(HH1)%202008/HH1%20Final %20v1.pdf (accessed 4 September 2009).

Pavolini, E. and Ranci, C. (2008), Restructuring the welfare state: reforms in long-term care in Western European countries, *European Journal of Social Policy*, 18, 3: 246–59.

Philpott, T. (ed.) (2008), *Residential Care: A Positive Future*, New Malden: Residential Forum.

Pickard, L. (1999), Policy options for informal carers of elderly people. In *With Respect to Old Age: Long Term Care – Rights and Responsibilities*, Research Vol. 3 of the Report of the Royal Commission on Long Term Care, Cm 4192-II/3, London: Stationery Office.

Pickard, L. (2001), Carer break or carer blind? Policies for informal carers in the UK, *Social Policy & Administration*, 35, 4: 441–58.

Pickard, L., Wittenberg, R., Comas-Herrera, A., Davies, B. and Darton, R. (2000), Relying on informal care in the new century? Informal care for elderly people in England to 2031, *Ageing and Society*, 20: 745–72.

Pickard, L., Wittenberg, R., Comas-Herrera, A., King, D. and Malley, J. (2007), Care by spouses, care by children: projections of informal care for older people in England to 2031, *Social Policy and Society*, 6, 3: 353–66.

Royal Commission on Long Term Care (1999), *With Respect to Old Age*, Cm 4192, London: Stationery Office.

Samuel, M. (2009), Direct payments, personal budgets and individual budgets: expert guides, *Community Care* (8 April 2009). Available at: www.communitycare.co.uk/ Articles/2009/04/08/102669/direct-payments-personal-budgets-and-individual-budgets.htm.

Scope (2009), Shaping the future of care together – Green Paper July 2009: A reaction from Scope, *Scope Update* (August 2009). Available at: ctt-news.org/6J4-1MD7-09Q05BS78/cr.aspx (accessed 4 September 2009).

Secretary of State for Health (2000), *The NHS Plan: The Government's Response to the Royal Commission on Long Term Care*, Cm 4818-II, London: Stationery Office.

6, P. (2003), Giving consumers of British public services more choice: what can be learned from recent history? *Journal of Social Policy*, 32, 2: 239–70.

Wanless, D., Forder, J., Fernandez, J.-L., Poole, T., Beesley, L., Henwood, M. and Moscone, F. (2006), *Securing Good Care for Older People: Taking a Long-term View*, London: King's Fund.

3

Reforming Long-term Care Policy in France: Private–Public Complementarities

Blanche Le Bihan and Claude Martin

Introduction

The definition of a specific long-term care (LTC) policy – or, to use French terminology, a policy for the 'dependent elderly' – really emerged at the end of the 1980s and has evolved progressively until today. It has been a long process, and one which will still be open to different scenarios over the next few years. The French LTC system cuts across many different sectors as it is fragmented between health insurance, domiciliary care and residential social care, state support through tax deductions for families who employ a carer and 'cash for care' benefits for the frail elderly, a large-scale private insurance sector, not to mention the crucial contribution of informal caregivers within families. Still, since the end of the 1990s, public sector participation in the financing and provision of LTC has been mainly organized around a 'dependency allowance'. After a period of local experimentation (1995–6), public policy has consisted mostly of a 'cash-for-care' scheme, initially targeting the more dependent and economically disadvantaged, and made available to all frail elderly people in 2002. The 2002 reform, which created the *Allocation personnalisée à l'autonomie* (APA), was the main turning-point in policy-framing. The number of people receiving the benefit rose from 150,000 in December 2001 to 1.115 million in December 2008, exceeding the number of dependent elderly estimated in 1999 by the first national inquiry (*Handicap, incapacité, dépendance*) of the National Institute of Statistics (INSEE).

As in other countries, the French LTC policy is facing financial constraints, exacerbated by the current financial crisis. Common exposure to funding pressures could be one of the main arguments to defend the hypothesis of European convergence, as all systems in Europe are becoming progressively mixed, combining informal care, assistance, national and private insurance, commodified and public services; in other words, they are based on a complex combination of family, market and state.

This chapter presents the policy-framing process, which began in the 1980s and has led to the so-called 'French compromise' (Le Bihan and Martin 2007), combining elements of different types of care system. We argue that the

French LTC system is in permanent evolution and can be analysed in terms of policy-learning, based on the successive adjustments of the system to adapt it to the evolution of the increasing demand on one side and the decreasing financial resources on the other side. This policy is a good example of path dependence of the French welfare system. Evidence from France suggests that LTC reform can only take place from the combination of public and private support, conceived as complementary.

We will first present the different components of this policy, based on both public and private supports, as well as its overall cost, and then focus on its core, i.e. the cash-for-care allowance created at the end of the 1990s and intended for old dependent people. In the discussion, we shall analyse the last phase of this policy framing: since the last presidential election in May 2007, a new direction towards an insurance model has been announced. But what does this mean in practice? What type of insurance model is proposed? The reform has not been implemented yet and many professional and social partners are worried about this delay and the practical aspects of this project of reform, which would appear to be a new compromise between the three poles of protection: the family, the market, and the state.

A Fragmented Policy

Confronted by the ageing of its population, France has, over the last few decades, developed a specific LTC policy for the elderly. The objective is to complement the informal care provided by relatives (mainly women), which still represents the main contribution to the provision of the care needs of the elderly. The LTC system does not constitute a homogeneous policy field. It cuts across a range of policies in the public sector such as social care, health care, family, employment and old age. To identify the many financial sources and the overall cost of such a fragmented policy, a distinction must be made between the public policy core, based on a specific LTC scheme – the *Allocation personnalisée d'autonomie* (APA) – created in 2002 to meet the needs of the frail elderly, private health insurance contributions, and more peripheral measures, which do not specifically concern elderly people but have an important impact on this policy sector.

Priority to home care and the risk of care deficit

As in many European countries, helping the elderly to live at home is presented as a priority in France (Martin 2003). The objective is both to contain the cost of the care system, as care in residential homes appears to be very expensive, and to satisfy the wish of many elderly people to continue living at home for as long as possible. Indeed, more than 90 per cent of people aged 75 and over live at home, and three out of four aged over 85 (FNORS 2008).[1] But who takes care of these elderly people at home? Estimates (DREES 2009) show that in France, 75 per cent of the dependent elderly in need of care receive support from relatives, who on average spend twice as much time with their parents than professionals. Half of primary informal carers are spouses (the wife in two-thirds of cases), while a third are daughters and sons (daughters in every three out of four cases). The average age of these family carers is 71 for spouses and 55 for children. In fact, 80 per cent of primary carers are aged between 50 and 79 (Dutheil 2001).

According to European statistical projections made in the research programme FELICIE (Future Elderly Living Conditions in Europe) (Gaymu 2008; Gaymu *et al.* 2008), 'on average, the disabled elderly of the future will be better equipped than those of today, both personally – because of higher levels of education – and socially, because they will be more frequently supported by their spouse and, at least potentially, by their children' (Gaymu *et al.* 2008: 257). Informal support from spouses has always been very much gender-based. In 2000, the majority of dependent men had the support of a partner or a child (53 per cent), while it was the case for only 16 per cent of women. Over the next few decades, this situation will evolve, with a new generation of parents reaching old age. Moreover, with the decrease in mortality and the reduction of the difference in life expectancy between men and women, widowhood will decrease, and partners will grow old together. For all these reasons, lack of family support could be less frequent, and 'the increased number of spouses as primary informal caregivers will generally be husbands rather than wives' (2008: 262).

Nevertheless, in spite of these changes, the risk of a care deficit remains high: first, because 'disabled people living with a partner will, on average, be older than they are today' (Gaymu *et al.* 2008: 265), which means that spouses as potential carers will themselves frequently be disabled; and second, because we do not know the future degree of family involvement in care tasks. Changes in women's employment patterns need to be taken into account; these show that women are remaining in paid work for longer and are confronted with the difficulties of combining work and family, even as senior workers (Le Bihan and Martin 2008). The increase in the number of divorces is another important variable. The problem, therefore, is not that of the potential of family carers, but of their availability and their desire to invest themselves in care tasks. These various elements clearly indicate the risk of a care deficit that will have to be addressed by both public policy and families, and the crucial need to invest in policies to support informal carers over the next few decades.

The cost of public LTC policy

The core of the French LTC policy is based on a specific allowance, the *Allocation personnalisée à l'autonomie*, distributed and managed at a local level (the French *Départements*). Amounting to nearly €5 billion, the allowance is mainly and increasingly covered by local taxes (up to 68 per cent in 2008). Only a complement is transferred by the state (table 1).

However, the public cost of 'dependency' is also supported by other measures, which do not specifically concern the elderly. The major contribution of the social security system should be taken into consideration; this pays hospitals and medical costs for the elderly, health costs in residential homes and for nursing at home, and represents almost €13 billion. Paradoxically, the main cost does not correspond to the core of the policy, but to the expenses related to the health-care system due to the care needs of the frail elderly.

The tax deduction policy,[2] implemented at the end of the 1990s to reduce the cost of home-care services and to develop employment in this sector of activity, is another measure which contributes to the funding of LTC policy (€387 million). Finally, the familial and retirement branches of the social security system are also concerned, paying €568 and €370 million, respectively (Vasselle 2008).

The overall public cost for the dependent elderly in 2008 was around €21 billion (60 per cent of which corresponds to the health-care social security cost) (Vasselle 2008: 17), representing a little over 1 per cent of GDP, more or less the same as in the UK or Germany, but half the cost in the USA or in Scandinavian countries. Estimations for the next 20 to 25 years are that the overall cost of LTC policies in France could reach 2.0–2.5 per cent of GDP.

A fragmented supply of health care and social services

The various public measures related to LTC concern two types of care: home-based and residential care. To support families in their care tasks, the elderly may resort to professional services, from both the health and social sectors. Nurses and nursing care attendants (aides soignantes), either independent workers or from non-profit-making organizations (SSIAD, services de soins infirmiers à domicile – 'nursing services at home'), are the main health professionals. They visit the elderly person at home and deliver personal and medical care (medicine, personal hygiene, etc.). The problem is the shortage of such services, funded by the social security and therefore free for the user. In 2007 there were 2,000 SSIAD offering 88,000 places, only 1.8 places for every 100 people aged 75 and above (FNORS 2008). The policy towards the frail elderly has also developed professional social-care services. These services

Table 1

APA expenditures

	2002	2003	2004	2005	2006	2007	2008
Number of recipients	605,000	792,000	865,000	938,000	1,008,000	1,070,000	1,100,000
Global cost (million €)	1,855	3,205	3,632	3,900	4,243	4,600	4,900
Local authorities (departments)	1,405	2,002	2,292	2,559	2,832	3,149	3,346
State	798	1,323	1,339	1,341	1,411	1,451	1,554
Local authorities' contribution (%)	57	58.7	63.1	65.88	66.75	68.46	68.29

Source: Vasselle (2008).

are provided by public structures or non-profit-making organizations, offering cleaning services as well as personal assistants to care for the elderly. However, the provision of home-care services is organized at a local level, with a limited availability of resources, and a degree of regional inequality. The payment of such services is reliant on families and on the specific cash allowance – the APA.

When home-based care is no longer possible, the elderly person may turn to residential care. At the beginning of 2006, there were 669,000 places in residential care and 10,000 residential homes for the elderly (FNORS 2008), organized as follows: 435,000 places in nursing homes, 153,000 in collective housing *(foyer logement)*, 72,400 in long-term care hospital services *(unités de soins de longue durée)* and 7,800 in temporary housing (FNORS 2008). Since 2002, institutions for the dependent elderly have been reorganized, and a unique category grouping the different institutions devoted to the dependent elderly has been created: the *EHPAD* *(établissement d'hébergement pour personnes âgées dépendantes,* 'institutions for the dependent elderly). The funding of these LTC institutions is based on three elements: accommodation, the cost of which – paid by the elderly person and their family – varies from institution to institution, or, in situations of low income, through social assistance; costs related to dependency, paid by the APA and the resident; and health-care costs, covered by social health insurance.

The private LTC system

With about 3 million policy-holders – totalling €2.1 billion in 2007 – France is proportionally the largest private insurance market in this field, ahead of the USA (with approximately 7 million policy-holders for a population which is 5 times greater). Nevertheless, compared to the 14 million people over 60 in France, it remains a small proportion of the potential market (Kessler 2008; Dufour-Kippelen 2008; De Castries 2009).

This market began to develop in the mid-1980s, and offers a variety of products, both individual and collective, which guarantee a monthly cash benefit in the event of dependency. In the USA, private insurance policies provide the reimbursement of care and service costs generated by dependency, which is not an easy system to monitor given the uncertainty of the level of reimbursement. It is indeed difficult to anticipate the level of dependency and therefore the level and cost of the needs (Taleyson 2007). In contrast, the French system is based on a fixed-sum payment, which is also much more flexible, allowing policy-holders to choose the organization of care and services as they wish. Four main types of contract are available:

- The *contrat de prévoyance* (contingency cover), where the policy-holder pays a regular premium in order to receive a predefined benefit in the event of dependency. If the risk does not occur, the global amount of cumulated premium is lost.
- An option in the life insurance policy, which gives the possibility of receiving the death or retirement pay-out in advance in the event of dependency.

- The *contrats d'épargne dépendance assurance-vie* (life insurance and dependency cover), in which the policy-holder can cumulate savings on their policy and can choose to convert them to a monthly benefit in the event of dependency. The policy-holders do not lose their savings.
- The *contrat complémentaire santé* (additional health cover), which is an option in private health insurance policies.

These insurance policies may be individual or collective (when an enterprise, mutual insurance company or a non-profit-making organization is the contractor), and when they are collective they may be either optional or compulsory.

The development of this private sector is linked to the real cost of dependency and the difficulty in covering these costs. To give an idea of the gap between public support and actual costs, here are some general estimates: dependency generates an average monthly cost of €2,500 (and up to €3,500 for a high dependency level). The public allowance (APA) contributes about €500 (up to €800 for a very high level of dependency), given that the average pension is about €1,200 per month. Middle-income households suffer the most from this financial situation, as the more disadvantaged households may rely entirely on public support and the more wealthy are able to use their own economic resources. Private insurance contributes an additional €300 on average. This figure means that a high level of dependency requires elderly people to use their savings, reducing what they are able to leave in inheritance and often meaning they must sell their home to pay for the services. They often fall into debt through meeting these costs, and this situation could deteriorate in the near future due to demographic pressure. As Courbage and Roudaut 2008: 645) put it: 'Low rates of public LTC coverage suggest that the financial consequences of dependency could be catastrophic, even resulting in ruin, for a number of elderly people and their families.'

Courbage and Roudaut studied the main obstacles to the development of this private market in France. They tested the main hypotheses: lack of information for potential users, moral hazard (defined as the over-consumption encouraged by insurance coverage), adverse selection (over-representation of high risk in the insured population), and the fact that public cover crowds out private insurance. Some of these analyses have been confirmed: people who have been confronted by disability, dependency, chronic disease or serious illness are more aware of these risks and more often purchase private insurance. Adverse selection also plays a role, as high-risk individuals also tend to take out such insurance policies more frequently. However, they also discovered that in France 'LTC insurance is strongly driven by altruistic behaviours. It is purchased not only to preserve bequests and to financially protect family or relatives in the event of disability, but also to reduce the burden on potential informal caregivers' (2008: 647). This altruistic argument could be one of the main reasons to explain the development of these insurances and their take-up rate.

Thus, many experts – mainly those working in the field of private insurance – argue that a public–private partnership is necessary to face the increase of these costs in the near future.

Reforming the Pillar of the French System: The *Allocation Personnalisée d'Autonomie*

Considering the policies implemented in EU countries, two types of systems can be identified (Costa-Font and Font-Vilalta 2006): contributory systems, based on social insurance – the German LTC insurance – and non-contributory systems, based on taxation – which exist in the Nordic countries as well as in Italy. Following this second logic at first, the French allowance appears today as a mix of the two systems, combining taxation and social contribution.

The development of a policy based on cash-for-care: a slow process

In France, the development of a policy regarding the dependent elderly has been a very slow process. As already mentioned, it appeared on the political agenda in the mid-1980s, but until 1994 there was no specific public LTC policy, only an in-depth political debate and numerous expert reports (Kessler 1994; Martin 2003). Until the mid-1990s, the main social-care policy for the frail elderly was in fact the same as that for the disabled: the *Allocation compensatrice pour tierce personne* (ACTP) ('compensatory allowance for a third party'), created in 1975, which had been extended to the elderly. The debate on LTC public policy centred on the idea of the creation of a specific cash benefit, attributed to elderly people suffering from physical and mental incapacity and requiring help in the activities of day-to-day life. This cash-for-care orientation, which is a common trend in various European countries (Da Roit *et al.* 2007), also supports recourse to informal and formal care, cost containment, and choice for users (Ungerson and Yeandle 2007). Conceived as a complement to family care, and presented as a financial support to outsource part of care activities and to purchase services, cash-for-care schemes involve major personal investment from family carers, in the role of care managers. Family carers set up a care arrangement, have regular contacts with the social and health professionals needed, and manage all the administrative part.

During the 1980s and 1990s, the definition of this cash-for-care orientation raised important issues. The first of these was the choice between social insurance and social assistance (Frinault 2003). The social insurance model was defended in one of the first official reports in 1979 (Arreckx 1979), but since then, very few experts – at least until 2007 – have supported the scenario of dependency as a fifth social security risk.[3] The second issue was whether the scheme should be universal or – in the logic of social assistance – whether it should concern only old people unable to pay for services. This principle has major consequences in terms of family obligations. In France there is a legal obligation (*obligation alimentaire*) for intergenerational solidarity (both upwards and downwards), imposing the support of relatives. The application of such a principle can mean that public cover is secondary to family support. The third issue was how the policy should be funded and managed, and to what extent the state, local authorities and social security funds should be involved. One of the main obstacles was financial. In the context of budgetary constraints, with a policy of curbing public expenditure, it was difficult to promote a policy for which the cost had not been properly estimated. At that time, even the number of dependent elderly people and potential recipients was unknown. The selection of a social insurance scheme was therefore considered as inappropriate and involving a too great risk of social security deficit.

These challenges, and the government's difficulty in facing these uncertainties, may explain the slowness of the decision-making process. Since the mid-1990s, four steps can be identified in the creation of a specific public long-term care scheme and the progressive increase in the number of recipients (Martin 2001). In 1994–5, an experimental pilot scheme developed by some local authorities (12 *Départements*) was put into practice. The objective was to enable local actors to develop their own scheme and experiment with the possibilities of creating a specific long-term care allowance. Then, in 1997, a temporary national assistance scheme, the *Prestation spécifique dépendance* (PSD), was implemented at a local level. The logic of assistance was threefold: to reduce public costs, to maintain family obligations, and to focus on the more disadvantaged and dependent elderly. The benefit – both means- and needs-tested – granted to dependent elderly people at home and in institutions, was very limited. It excluded average dependency, which represented almost 40 per cent of all recipients and people on middle incomes. The possibility of recovering funds from the elderly person's estate also excluded a large share of recipients, as most families wanted to preserve their inheritance. The cost containment objective was therefore reached and families remained the main carers.

However, the many criticisms of this scheme – particularly the fact that in 2001 only 15 per cent of frail elderly people received the benefit (150,000 recipients) – made a reform of the care system necessary. The aim of the 2002 socialist reform was clear: to move away from the PSD scheme and to increase the number of recipients. The policy shifted from a logic of assistance to universalism, with the implementation of the *Allocation personnalisée à l'autonomie*, allocated to elderly people with high and middle levels of dependency, and attributed in proportion to the level of income and without the possibility of claiming from inheritance (see details below).

The next step occurred in 2004, after the heatwave of summer 2003,[4] the consequences of which demonstrated the need to combine formal and informal sources of support, and to facilitate the connection between health care and social services. It revealed the importance of local response to such crises and the need for the administrative authorities to prepare for such events. In terms of policy-framing, however, this tragedy has forced decision-makers to make some significant changes. Although even before the heatwave the government considered the possibility of reducing the public cost of the APA scheme, the orientation changed, and an alternative to retrenchment was proposed. In this new context, the 1995 German reform, introducing a LTC social insurance (Geraedts *et al.* 2000; see also Rothgang, this volume), was presented as a model.

The summer 2003 tragedy led the government to adopt new measures with the organization of a 'Plan for the Dependent Elderly' (a first Plan was implemented for the period 2004–7, and a second for the period 2008–12). Three main elements were introduced: a programme to deal with any future

Table 2

CNSA expenses in 2008 (€)

	Elderly dependent people	Disabled people
Support to individuals	1.6 billion	596 million
Institutions and services	6.1 billion	7.7 billion
Specific fundings	77 million to specific actions (innovations and professionalization) in both sectors 22 million to prevention and studies in both sectors	

Source: See: http://cnsa.fr.

heatwave,[5] an improvement in the epidemiological warning system and, in 2005, a specific Fund for the frail elderly and disabled people (the *Caisse nationale de solidarité pour l'autonomie* – CNSA). In the same way as the German insurance scheme, this new fund is financed by an employer contribution[6] in return for the suppression of one day of public holiday,[7] an additional contribution (0.3 per cent on financial and property holdings) and 0.1 per cent of the *Contribution Sociale Généralisée* (CSG) (tax principle), and the transfer of credits devoted to elderly and disabled people in the social security fund. This fund – which represented €15 billion in 2008 (Vasselle 2008): 12.6 billion transferred from health insurance and 2.4 billion provided by the specific tax and the employers' contribution – was presented as a step towards the social insurance principle. Covering both disabled people and elderly dependent people (table 2) the fund also marks the introduction of a new global conception of 'dependency'.

Main characteristics of the APA

The French APA scheme has three main features. First, it is a benefit given to elderly people whether living at home or in institutions[8] according to their level of dependency. The French system is based on a single assessment scale, the AGGIR,[9] which distinguishes six levels of dependency (from GIR1 (the highest) to GIR6): the APA is allocated up to the fourth level. Because the French scheme is a national one implemented at a local level, and in order to guarantee access to the same services across the country, each level of dependency gives entitlement to a capped amount of benefit. In January 2008, the amounts were the following: a maximum of €1,209 for GIR1, €1,036 for GIR2, €777 for GIR3 and €518 for GIR4.

Second – and this is a main characteristic of the French scheme – the benefit is paid to finance a specific care package determined by a team of professionals according to the needs of the recipient. The use of the benefit is controlled, and it can only finance care identified as necessary by professionals. The paid carers can either be professional workers, or relatives (except the

43

Table 3

Average amount of APA depending of the level of dependency

	Local authority contribution	Contribution of the recipient (and % of the recipients concerned by a co-payment)	Average amount
Average amount of APA at home (€)			
GIR1	833	174 (73%)	1,007
GIR2	635	149 (77%)	785
GIR3	474	104 (77%)	577
GIR4	289	59 (78%)	349
Total	*406*	*88 (78%)*	*494*
Amount in institution			
GIR1 and 2	396	151	547
GIR3 and 4	195	140	335
All	*313*	*146*	*460*

Source: DREES (2009).

spouse). The logic is therefore one of free choice – the family takes part in the choice of the care arrangement and can combine professional and family care – but the type of care needed is determined by professionals. This control of the benefit is an important feature of the scheme[10] and introduces a stronger regulation than in other European countries where cash-for-care has also been adopted (Glendinning 2006; Da Roit *et al.* 2007; Ungerson and Yeandle 2007).

Finally, France has adopted a twofold system to finance care packages. In the first instance, an 'assistance principle' is applied: below a fixed income threshold (€682), recipients do not contribute at all to the funding of the care package. In the second instance, a 'user fee' or co-payment system has been introduced: above the threshold, the recipient contributes to the financing of the care package according to this level of income. Thus all recipients can receive the APA allowance, but their contribution or co-payment varies according to their means (see table 3). Above a monthly income of €2,720 per month, the APA recipient pays 90 per cent of the care package.

The APA replaced the PSD in January 2002. It was highly successful, with a very rapid increase in the number of claimants. Between January 2002 and June 2003, some 1,390,000 people claimed the APA, and 723,000 people received it.[11] In December 2008, some 1,115,000 people received the APA. Statistics show that more dependent people are mainly cared for in institutions, while recipients with medium and medium-high dependency levels remain at home (table 4).

Discussion: Seeking Public/Private Complementarity

Until now, the development of each system – public and private – has been independent: private LTC cover was not conceived as a complement of public

Table 4

Number of APA recipients (thousands) according to level of
dependency, December 2008

	At home	In institution	All
GIR1	17	67	85
	2.5%	15.7%	7.6%
GIR2	124	184	307
	18%	43.1%	27.5%
GIR3	149	69	218
	21.7%	16.2%	19.6%
GIR4	399	106	505
	57.8%	25%	45.3%
Together	689	426	1,115
	100%	100%	100%

Source: DREES (2009).

cover as it is for the health system. Policy-holders invested in private insurance without knowing if the money received would be sufficient to pay for the difference between the amount of the LTC public allowance and the actual cost of the care needed.

Since the end of 2005, four major official reports have been published concerning the French LTC policy[12] and its future. The main challenge is the funding of the system, taking into account demographic and public-health estimates. The Ministry of Work and Social Affairs considers that the cost of the APA in 2040 will double and reach between €10 and €11.5 billion per year – compared to €4.7 billion in 2007. Moreover, 5,000 to 7,500 additional nursing home places will be needed per year. These growing requirements are challenging the system, and decision-makers have been looking for a solution. In this perspective, the balance of private/public cover is a main issue. The French LTC system offers two types of cover, both based on a 'lump sum' logic. The question now is that of their articulation: how can they be made to complement each another?

The social insurance model: political rhetoric?

Since the beginning of the policy process in the 1980s, French decision-makers have carefully examined the LTC social insurance model. Initially abandoned, this scenario is now regularly on the political agenda, as it is presented as a solution covering what is defined as the 'risk of dependency'. In this perspective, the government has on several occasions announced the creation of a 'fifth risk'. However, it is necessary to specify what this announcement means and what lies behind the 'insurance model'.

The implementation of the German LTC social insurance in the 1990s remains an example for French decision-makers. As already mentioned, confronted by the heatwave disaster of summer 2003, the French government has imported some characteristics of the German scheme: first, an insurance glossary – *caisse* (fund), *contribution* (social contribution), and *nouvelle branche de la protection sociale* (new branch of the social security system); second – in the same way as the German LTC social insurance scheme – a new employer social security contribution in return for one day of public holiday; and third, the creation of a new social fund (*caisse nationale de solidarité à l'autonomie* – CNSA).

However, these different elements do not mean that a social insurance framework has been implemented in France. The experience of the German LTC social insurance scheme reveals that the creation of a stabilized 'fifth risk' has not yet occurred (Taleyson 2007). Implemented in 1994, the German compulsory LTC insurance has shown the limits of this model. Based on social contribution – 1.7 per cent contribution by employees and employers – it has to face an important deficit, assessed as up to more than €800 million in 2006. To reduce this deficit, an increase of social contributions has been decided in 2008 (+0.25 per cent), but experts are worried about the durability of such a system. Estimates show that to cover the needs, social contribution will have to rise up to 3.5 per cent in 2030 and 6 per cent in 2050 (Taleyson 2007), which is very difficult to apply.

Considering the German experience and the weight of existing taxes in France, a compulsory public system based on an additional social contribution would appear difficult to develop (Albouy 2009). Thus, it is perfectly clear that the new fund (*caisse*) is quite different from the social security funds (*caisses de sécurité sociale*) already in existence in the fields of health, retirement or family: there are no representatives of social partners on the board (*conseil d'administration*) of the CNSA. The executive board is composed of representatives from the funding institutions – the state and local authorities – and representatives of the health branch of the social security system. A specific consultative board has also been set up (*conseil d'orientation et de surveillance*), associating representatives from private insurance companies, and non-profit-making organizations providing services. Thus, it is impossible to consider the French LTC system as a social insurance system.

It is interesting to note that the Spanish reform adopted in December 2006 raised similar problems and questions. A political orientation was first taken towards a social insurance system with the White Paper commissioned by the national ministry of employment and social affairs (*El Libro Blanco de la Dependencia*) and published in 2004. This White Paper argued that in order to move away from the assistance and familistic model, Spain had the choice between a universal socio-democratic route and a social insurance route. Considering that the conditions of the first model (universal access to services controlled by the state and professionalization of care) were out of reach in the Spanish case, the White Paper suggested promoting a social insurance model. Nevertheless, the Law adopted in December 2006 is far from these recommendations, due to the opposition of employers to covering these new costs and of the Autonomous Communities, who are also reluctant to incur such a loss of control in service provision. The difficulties of implementing such a LTC model led to a reorganization of the scheme, which may prove the existence of the strong inertia of a familistic regime (León 2009).

The question of the insurability of the risk of dependency is a main challenge in itself. The difficulty of foreseeing the evolution of the cost of long-term care is the first problem. Indeed, if an extension of life expectancy goes hand-in-hand with an extension of the period of life spent with a disability, there is a risk of escalating costs. However, it is very difficult to form a precise idea of this evolution. Some analyses show that, due to medical progress and quality of life, life expectancy without loss of autonomy is rising more rapidly. The next generation of elderly people will not have the same problems as previous generations. A recent report by the OECD concerning twelve countries (Lafortune and Balestat 2007) has even demonstrated that the risk of high dependency varies from country to country: it is diminishing in the USA, Denmark, Finland, the Netherlands and Italy, stable in Australia and Canada, and increasing in Japan, Belgium and Sweden. The data available do not allow an assessment of the evolution in France and the UK. This unpredictability of cost is a main obstacle to the development of a social insurance scheme. How can public authorities commit themselves to fully cover a risk that is impossible to anticipate?

The definition of dependency is a second problem. What does it mean in practice? How is it assessed? Do the public and private systems use the same tools to estimate dependency and/or needs? Dependency is a complex risk, due to several different factors: physical, mental, and also social. Defined as the inability to perform some of the most basic daily activities (getting up, washing, dressing, etc.) without third-party assistance, it is accentuated by social factors, such as the presence or absence of family support. The precise definition of the risk of dependency is presented by Durand and Taleyson (2003) as a main condition for the insurability of such a risk and to limit the uncertainty of funding. The two authors identify two types of approach. The first refers to 'care', which is defined as 'long-term' and is characteristic of the American (*long-term care*) or German (*Pflegeversicherung*) systems. The second approach – which is also the French approach – does not use the term 'care' (*soins*), but rather 'dependency' or 'loss of autonomy'. These notions do not refer to needs, but more to the physical, mental and social state of the elderly person, an approach which is said to facilitate the assessment of the situation. The national AGGIR grid sets out different acts of day-to-day life – to wake up, to get dressed, to wash oneself, to do the shopping, to cook, to move, etc. – and aims to define precisely the level of autonomy of the person assessed (she can completely, partially or not at all).

The latest reform proposal: the private/public balance

Another step forward was announced by the government of François Fillon after the last Presidential election in May 2007. This reform, based on the creation of a 'fifth risk' – dependency – was supposed to be implemented at the end of 2008, then delayed to 2009 and we are still waiting for the details at the time of writing (November 2009). However, it is possible to analyse the main orientations.

A report was published by the *Sénat* in July 2008 to prepare for this reform: *La prise en charge de la dépendance et la création du cinquième risque* ('Long-term care and the creation of the fifth risk'; Vasselle 2008). This 'fifth risk' refers directly to the French social protection system and corresponds, once again, to the social insurance glossary. On the website of the government, it is defined as follows: 'The fifth risk is a new field of the social security system. It will complement the existing ones covering health, family, pensions and work injuries. The fifth risk can also be named 'dependency risk' or 'risk of loss of autonomy'.[13]

However, the creation of a 'fifth risk', as proposed by the French government, is in fact a multi-pillar system, combining public cover and private insurance. The first pillar is based on the existing public system, with the APA and the fund (CNSA), and defends collective solidarity. It aims to guarantee all elderly dependent citizens universal access to a needs assessment and to a minimum care package allocated at a local level by the *Départements*. The second pillar formalizes the contribution of the recipient: in order to contain costs, the principle of 'recovery on inheritance' could be reintroduced: above a threshold yet to be defined (between €150,000 and €200,000) of total household capital, part of the amount of the APA delivered will be recovered on inheritance. An alternative is proposed: the recipients may choose to receive only 50 per cent of the APA allowance, without recovery on inheritance. In any case, this public cover is not and will not be sufficient to finance all the needs of the dependent elderly. As inheritance and bequests are very important in French culture, it is highly likely that families organize themselves to preserve it.

Recovery on inheritance was one of the criteria for obtaining the first allowance created in 1997 (PSD), and at that time, many elderly people were reluctant to ask for the allowance. The reintroduction of such criteria will probably have similar consequences, and other solutions therefore need to be proposed. This is precisely the objective of the French government's reform, which presents private insurance as the third pillar of the long-term care system. With up to 15 per cent of annual growth (Kessler 2008), private insurance is widespread in France. Based on a 'lump sum' logic, the French private system offers a precise definition of the risk of dependency. Instead of covering personal care needs, which are very difficult to anticipate, the insurers cover a specific state – a high-level and irreversible dependency – referring to Activities of Daily Living (ADLs) (Taleyson 2007). However, the sector remains marginal in comparison with the number of people concerned. The objective is to expand the private insurance market.

Different solutions have been suggested. The introduction of tax incentives to attract middle-income households is a first possibility, but the government's proposition goes further: without making insurance compulsory, the complementarity of public/private coverage proposed in the reform is a way to incite people to subscribe to private insurance policies. This combination of different solutions concerns not only public and private cover, but also private insurance and life insurance[14] and reverse mortgaging (Courbage 2009). A reverse mortgage is a bank loan guaranteed through property and used to enable elderly people to finance long-term care, without having to sell their homes. Some experts (Chen 2001) go even further and propose the development of reverse mortgaging in order to finance life or dependency insurance.

However, there are many obstacles to the development of such a system: it is open only to home-owners and even then it is not an attractive solution, as it could mean the end of succession (Assier-Andrieu and Gotman 2009).

This controversial proposition has already provoked many comments and reactions. The socialist party and the main left-wing social partners consider it as a deception which implies a major social regression. A truly new field of social protection should be based on wider collective solidarity, on higher taxation and social security contributions. It should also involve a new system of representation on the Board of the CNSA, etc. The critics also underline the fact that the cost of such a system will weigh heavily on middle-income households, with a low threshold to activate recovery on inheritance (€150,000 or €200,000 of household capital). Finally, this project of reform is considered as a Trojan horse in the social security system: a step forward towards a dual and liberal model.

In addition to this, reactions from social and professional partners of the sector (such as the *Union nationale des centres communaux d'action sociale*, the *Association des paralysés de France*, the *Fédération nationale des accidents du travail et des handicapés*, the *Union nationale de l'aide*, etc.) are negative. Most of them consider that the reform will weaken the LTC scheme and the representation of users and citizens in the system. They would also prefer to develop a true social insurance scheme, with new collective contributions.

At the time of writing the original article preceding this chapter, we were still waiting for this main reform, which has been postponed due to the financial crisis, which certainly plays an important role in this attitude of waiting: 'The room to manoeuvre disappeared in the financial turmoil' (Vanackère 2009: 4). The government is aware of the political risk in rushing towards private insurance schemes, and many professional partners concerned (*Fédération française des sociétés d'assurance, Fédération nationale des mutuelles de France, Caisse nationale de prévoyance*, etc.) are criticizing the project. The recent announcement of the reduction in resources for public nursing homes in order to contain the public cost of the system has aggravated the situation.

What Do We Learn from the French Case?

This chapter has sought to examine the source of reform of the LTC financing and organization in France. We have argued that the French policy remains open to different scenarios and major tensions, and this is one main characteristic of the reform process in France. Reform in France is characterized by evolution rather than change, and the former takes place by not making over-radical choices and preferring new compromises. Reform in France shows a close influence by the German reform, and particularly issues regarding the maintenance of a social insurance model based on a scenario of entitlement to care, which has many supporters. Policy developments suggest that there will be no creation of a new field of social protection like that of family, health or retirement; the logic is to promote complementarity and better coordination between private and public insurance. As the government does not want to increase either social contributions on wages or taxes, the only possibility is to develop private insurance schemes for those who can, and, for those who cannot, to propose services and a cash allowance with high limits: the obligation for the recipients to 'choose' a flat-rate minimum allowance, or to accept recovery on inheritance. Such a reform could produce a dual system of protection, with no 'genuine choice'. The public/private coverage balance is today's main challenge. The French policy process reveals the importance of the initial choices that were made in the 1990s: adoption of a cash-for-care public system, giving up of a traditional new social security branch, and addition of new sources of funding to make the system sustainable in the long run. All these elements, which remain today despite regular adjustments and reforms, confirm the path dependence of the French LTC policy.

Notes

1. Census 1999.
2. In France, when one has an employee at home (house cleaning, caring for the children, caring for the frail elderly) one is granted a tax relief of 50 per cent of the costs linked to this employment (wages, social charges).
3. The French social security system is based on four risks: illness, retirement, family and accident at work.
4. Some 15,000 elderly people died during this heatwave.
5. Air conditioning in retirement homes and hospitals, recruitment of professionals.
6. Called *Contribution solidarité autonomie*.
7. Called *journée de solidarité*.
8. In the case of institutions, the benefit can either be allocated to individuals or globally to the institution itself, which uses it according to the dependency needs of the residents. The choice between the two options is made by the institution. In France, institutions for the elderly distinguish three expenditure components: dependency costs (paid by the resident and the APA), accommodation costs (paid by the resident), and health-care costs (paid by through health insurance).
9. AGGIR means *Autonomie gérontologique et groupes iso-ressources*.
10. Administrative control is organized by local authorities and may vary from one *Département* to another.
11. This success also had an impact on the local and national political debate after the political change of April 2002 with the return of a Conservative government. The new government and right-wing local authorities criticized the escalating costs and the previous socialist government's failure to plan the funding of their care system for dependent elderly people. In April 2003, the decision was taken to lower the threshold under which recipients do not contribute to the funding of the care package, from €943 to €623 per month. This reform has reinforced the co-payment system by increasing the user's contribution and has contained costs.
12. Cour des Comptes (2005); CAS (2006); Gisserot and Grass (2007); Vasselle (2008).
13. Available at: http://premier-ministre.gouv.fr/information/questions_reponses_484/est_cinquiemerisque.
14. Some 12.5 million people have a life insurance policy such as this, representing 40 per cent of households to a total amount of €1,100 billion in 2007.

References

Albouy, F.-X. (2009), Y a-t-il une économie de la dépendance? [Is there an economics of dependency?], *Risques*, 78: 88–93.

Arreckx, M. (1979), *L'amélioration de la qualité de vie des personnes âgées dépendantes* [Improvement in the quality of life of dependent elderly people], Paris: La documentation française.

Assier-Andrieu, L. et Gotman, A. (2009), *Réversion du principe du logement humain: Chronique du prêt hypothécaire inversé* [Reversion of the principle of human housing: history of reverse mortgages], Rapport de recherche pour le Ministère du logement et le Ministère de l'écologie, de l'énergie, du développement durable et de l'aménagement du territoire, Document de travail Cerlis, Université de Paris Descartes, janvier 2009, 360 pages.

Centre d'analyse stratégique (CAS) (2006), *Personnes âgées dépendantes: bâtir le scénario du libre choix* [Frail elderly people: elaborating the free choice scenario], Paris: CAS.

Chen Y. P (2001), Funding long term care in the United States: the role of private insurance, *The Geneva Papers on Risk Insurance–Issue and Practice*, 26: 656–66.

Cour des Comptes (2005), *Les personnes âgées dépendantes* [Dependent elderly people], Rapport au Président de la République. Documentation française (November).

Courbage, C. (2009), La couverture du risque dépendance [The coverage of risk of dependency], *Risques*, 78: 107–13.

Courbage, C. and Roudaut, N. (2008), Empirical evidence on long-term care insurance purchase in France, *The Geneva Papers*, 33: 645–58.

Costa-Font, J. and Font-Vilalta, M. (2006), Design limitations of long-term care insurance schemes: a comparative study of the situation in Spain, *International Social Security Review*, 59, 4: 91–110.

Da Roit, B., Le Bihan, B. and Österle, A. (2007), Long term care reforms in Italy, Austria and France: variations in cash-for-care schemes, *Social Policy & Administration*, 41, 6: 653–71.

De Castries, H. (2009), Ageing and long-term care: key challenges in long-term care coverage for public and private systems, *The Geneva Papers*, 34: 24–34.

DREES (2009), L'allocation personnalisée d'autonomie et la prestation de compensation du handicap au 30 décembre 2008 [APA and the benefit for the handicapped on 30 December 2008], *Etudes et Résultats*, 690, 4 pages.

Dufour-Kippelen, S. (2008), *Les contrats d'assurance dépendance sur le marché français en 2006* [Dependency insurance contracts on the French market in 2006], DREES, Série Etudes et recherches, 84, 39 pages.

Dutheil, N. (2001), Les aides et les aidants des personnes âgées [Help and carers of elderly people], *Etudes et Résultats*, 142, 12 pages.

Durand, R. and Taleyson, L. (2003), Les raisons du succès de l'assurance dépendance en France [Reasons for the success of dependency insurance in France], *Risques*, 55 (September): 115–20.

FNORS (Fédération nationale des observatoires régionaux de la santé) (2008), *Vieillissement des populations et état de santé dans les régions de France* [The ageing of populations and state of health in the regions of France], Rapport de la FNORS (September).

Frinault, T. (2003), L'hypothèse du 5ème risque [The hypothesis of the fifth risk]. In C. Martin (ed.), *La dépendance des personnes âgées: Quelles politiques en Europe?* Rennes: Presses Universitaires de Rennes/Edition de l'ENSP, pp. 69–92.

Gisserot, H. and Grass, E. (2007), *Perspectives financières de la dépendance des personnes âgées à l'horizon 2025: prévisions et marges de choix* [Financial perspectives of frail elderly people to the year 2025: predictions and scope for choice], Rapport remis à M. P. Bas, Ministre délégué à la sécurité sociale, aux personnes âgées, aux personnes handicapées et à la famille (March), Paris: La Documentation française.

Gaymu, J. (2008), Comment les personnes dépendantes seront-elles entourées en 2030? Projections européennes [How will dependent people be supported in 2030? European forecasts], *Population et Sociétés*, Ined, 444.

Gaymu, J., Festy, P., Poulain, M. and Beets, G. (2008), *Future Elderly Living Conditions in Europe*, Paris: Institut national d'études démographiques.

Geraedts, M., Heller, G. V. and Harrington, C. A. (2000), Germany's long term care insurance: putting a social insurance model into practice, *Milbank Quarterly*, 78, 3: 375–401.

Glendinning, C. (2006), Paying family caregivers: evaluating different models. In C. Glendinning and P. Kemp (eds), *Cash and Care: Policy Challenges in the Welfare State*, Bristol: Policy Press, pp. 127–40.

Kessler, F. (1994), *La dépendance des personnes âgées, un défi pour le droit de la protection sociale* [The dependency of elderly people, a challenge for the right to social security], Actes du colloque du Centre de recherche de droit social de l'Université Robert Schuman, Strasbourg: Presses Universitaires de Strasbourg.

Kessler, D. (2008), The long-term care insurance market, *The Geneva Papers*, 33: 33–40.

Lafortune, G. and Balestat, G. (2007), *Trends in Severe Disability among Elderly People: Assessing the Evidence in 12 OECD Countries and the Future Implication*, OECD Health Working Paper, Paris: OECD.

Le Bihan, B. and Martin, C. (2007), Cash-for-care in the French welfare state: a skilful compromise? In C. Ungerson and S. Yeandle (eds), *Cash-for-care Systems in Developed Welfare States*, London: Palgrave, pp. 32–59.

Le Bihan, B. and Martin, C. (2008), Caring for dependent elderly parents and family configurations. In R. Jallinova and E. Widmer (eds), *Beyond the Nuclear Family: Families in a Configurational Perspective*, Frankfurt am Main: Peter Lang, pp. 57–74.

León, M. (2009), Recent developments in long-term care in the Spanish welfare state: restructuring 'familistic' practices. Working Paper presented at the 7th ESPAnet Conference, Urbino, 17–19 September.

Martin, C. (2001), Les politiques de prise en charge des personnes âgées dépendantes [Long-term care policies towards the frail elderly], *Travail, Genre et Sociétés*, 6: 83–103.

Martin, C. (ed.) (2003), *La dépendance des personnes âgées: Quelles politiques en Europe?* [Long-term care policies towards elderly people: which policies in Europe?], Rennes: Presses Universitaires de Rennes/Edition de l'ENSP.

Taleyson, L. (2007), L'enjeu de la définition de la dépendance: une comparaison internationale [The stakes in the definition of dependency: an international comparison], *Risques*, 72 (December): 28–35.

Vasselle, A. (2008), *Rapport d'information sur la prise en charge de la dépendance et la création du cinquième risque* [Report on long-term care towards elderly people and the creation of the fifth risk], Rapport au Sénat, annexe au procès verbal de la séance du 8 juillet 2008.

Ungerson, C. and Yeandle, S. (2007), *Cash-for-care Systems in Developed Welfare States*, London: Palgrave.

Vanackère, C. (2009), Dépendance, les clés pour comprendre le retard [Dependency: keys to understanding the delay], *Espace Social Européen*, 893 (April): 4–5.

4

Sustainability of Comprehensive Universal Long-term Care Insurance in the Netherlands

Frederik T. Schut and Bernard van den Berg

Introduction

In many OECD countries public expenditures on health and long-term care (LTC) are a matter of great concern in view of an ageing population and increasing constraints on public budgets. These concerns are particularly vexing for countries with relatively high public expenditures on LTC, such as the Netherlands. In comparison to most other OECD countries, both total and public expenditures on LTC in the Netherlands are high, particularly since the percentage of elderly people is similar to the OECD average (OECD 2005). This can at least partly be explained by the relatively generous social health insurance scheme.

Nevertheless, the growth of public spending on health and long-term care in the Netherlands was quite successfully limited until 2000 via the implementation of cost-containment policies. These policies acted essentially through the rationing of supply, wage moderation, price controls and postponement of investment in LTC facilities. However, increasing waiting lists and rising consumer expectations about the quality and variety of LTC services have substantially reduced the scope for containing LTC expenditures along these lines. Hence, the Dutch government is aiming to reform the current long-term care financing system to increase incentives for efficiency and consumer direction.

The main aims of this chapter are (1) to describe the background, past experience and proposals to reform the system of LTC financing in the Netherlands; and (2) to discuss whether the proposed reforms can create incentives to keep the comprehensive LTC insurance scheme sustainable in view of the ageing of the population and the expected increase in demand for LTC services.

The second section provides a short background of the Dutch public health insurance scheme. In the following section we discuss the main features of the current public insurance scheme, before analysing the empirical evidence on the growth of public expenditure on LTC over the period 1985–2005. The subsequent section describes the relation between professional and informal care, before focusing specifically on the implications of the introduction of the personal care budgets for the provision of informal care. Next we discuss the projections and determinants of future long-term expenditure growth. The following section discusses the shortcomings of the current system of long-term care financing, and then the proposals for reforming the system. Finally, we discuss the prospects of the reform and the questions that remain to be answered.

Since a uniform definition is lacking, we will first indicate what we mean by long-term care. Often LTC is used only in the context of elderly care. In this article, however, we use a more comprehensive definition, including also care for the mentally and physically handicapped and care for chronic psychiatric patients. This definition coincides with the types of services covered by the public insurance scheme for long-term care in the Netherlands.

Background of Public LTC Insurance

The Netherlands was the first country to introduce a universal mandatory social health insurance scheme (the Exceptional Medical Expenses Act, abbreviated as AWBZ) for covering a broad range of LTC services provided in a variety of care settings. Whereas in the Netherlands public LTC insurance had already been introduced in 1968, other countries followed only quite recently, like Germany in 1995 (see Rothgang, this volume) and Japan in 2000 (Ikegami 2007).

There are several reasons why in the Netherlands the choice was made for a separate universal public health insurance scheme for long-term care. First, prior to 1968 the financing of LTC facilities was highly fragmented and increasingly insufficient to provide access to adequate care for lower-income groups. The strong economic growth during the 1960s substantially increased the general welfare of society, but because of a lack of adequate funding the availability and quality of LTC facilities lagged behind this overall welfare increase. Hence, since the financial risk of LTC was considered to be largely uninsurable on a private market,[1] there was broad political support to expand public financing for it.

Second, because of the presence of a social health insurance scheme for curative health services (the Sickness Fund Act, abbreviated as ZFW) the choice was made for public insurance rather than tax financing (as, for instance, in Sweden and Norway). However, the prevailing sickness fund scheme covered only two-thirds of the population (primarily lower- and middle-income groups). Therefore, a straightforward expansion of this scheme by including long-term care in the mandatory benefits package was no option, because then the higher-income groups would not be included and would not have to contribute to the financing of long-term care. An option would have been to expand the prevailing mandatory social health insurance scheme from two-thirds to the entire population, alongside an expansion of the benefits package to include long-term care. Although this option was seriously considered and actually proposed by the government, the proposal was soon withdrawn because of strong resistance from private health insurers (fearing a substantial loss of business), employers (fearing increasing employer contributions) and the medical profession (fearing government control of fees for services to privately insured patients). Since an expansion of the prevailing social insurance scheme was not feasible (as, for instance, in Belgium and Switzerland), a separate mandatory insurance scheme for long-term care (AWBZ) for the entire Dutch population was proposed and enacted in 1968.

Initially, the AWBZ covered primarily nursing home care, institutionalized care for the mentally handicapped, and hospital admissions lasting more than a year. In due course, however, coverage was expanded by including home health care, e.g. for rehabilitation at home after hospital admission and care for elderly people with impairments (in 1980), ambulatory mental health care (in 1982), family care, e.g. home help in case of frailty, psychosocial problems or after childbirth (1989) and residential care for the elderly (1997). In homes for the elderly (residential care) residents receive nursing care less frequently and intensively than do residents in nursing homes. Moreover, residents in elderly homes have their own apartments, while residents in nursing homes usually share a room with one or more other residents.

Main Features of Public LTC Insurance

The AWBZ constitutes a mandatory insurance scheme for long-term care for the entire Dutch population. Every Dutch citizen older than 15 years of age with a taxable income has to pay an income-related contribution (up to a certain maximum amount) that is collected through the income and payroll tax systems, along with the contributions for the other national insurance schemes (e.g. for unemployment and disability). In addition, for most LTC services covered by the AWBZ, income-related co-payments are required. For higher-income groups the maximum co-payment can be so high (about €1,800 per month for residential care) that private facilities are often more attractive. Income-related contributions and co-payments, as well as an annual state subsidy are collected in a General Fund (abbreviated as AFBZ).

Table 1 provides an overview of the different sources of funding of the AWBZ in 2008. Since in the same year the total expenditures from the General Fund were €21.4 billion, there was an overall deficit of €2.1 billion (to be compensated by an extra increase in the 2009 contribution rate). As shown in table 1, more than 75 per cent of the AWBZ is financed directly by households, while the residual amount is paid by the state out of general taxes. Table 2 provides an overview of the most important categories of LTC users and their relative share in LTC expenditure.

Formally, the AWBZ is administered by health-care insurers which provide coverage for curative health services. In practice, however, health-care insurers have delegated various responsibilities – in particular the contracting of health-care providers, the collection of patient contributions and the organization of regional consultations – to the largest regional health-care insurer. At present, the Netherlands is divided into 32 care regions and in each region a single health insurer (known as 'regional care office') carries out the AWBZ on behalf of all health insurers for all residents living in that region. Regional care offices receive a fixed budget for the administrative tasks. All LTC expenses are directly paid out the General Fund (AFBZ). Hence, neither

Table 1

Funding of the AWBZ scheme in 2008

Sources of funding	Payments (billion euros)	Share of total payments (%)
Income-related contributions*	13.1	68
Co-payments	1.7	9
State subsidy (from general taxation)	4.6	24
Total	*19.3*	*100*

*In 2008 the income-related contribution was 12.15 per cent of a maximum of €31,589 taxable income (implying a maximum contribution of €3,838 per year, exclusive of various possible tax deductions).
Source: SER (2008: 31).

Table 2

Different groups of AWBZ beneficiaries by numbers and expenditures in 2007*

Type of LTC user	Number	Share of total number (%)	Expenditure (billion euro)	Share of total expenditure (%)
Elderly and chronically ill	360,000	69	11.4	65
Mentally handicapped persons	100,000	19	4.6	26
Physically handicapped persons	15,000	3	0.5	3
Chronic psychiatric patients	50,000	9	1.1	6
Total	*525,000*	*100*	*17.6*	*100*

*Excluding about 90,000 clients with a personal care budget (expenditure €1.3 billion).
Source: SER (2008: 34).

regional care offices nor individual health insurers are at risk for long-term care expenses covered by the AWBZ scheme.

Before a person can qualify for care under the AWBZ, it is necessary to establish whether care is really required and, if so, what type of care and how much care is needed. Initially, health-care providers were responsible for the required needs assessment, but in 1997 this task was assigned to regional independent needs assessment organizations, and since 2005 to a single national organization (the Centre for Needs Assessment, abbreviated as CIZ).[2] The idea behind this was to make needs assessment more objective and uniform, and independent from the self-interest of health-care providers. Notice that the access to LTC is solely based on a person's health – as in Germany and Japan – and does not depend on his/her income or wealth – like the Medicaid programme in the USA.[3]

Box 1

Functional categories of care covered by AWBZ

1. *Personal care*: e.g. help with taking a shower, bed baths, dressing, shaving, skin care, going to the toilet, eating and drinking.
2. *Nursing*: e.g. dressing wounds, giving injections, advising on how to cope with illness, showing clients how to self-inject.
3. *Supportive guidance*: e.g. helping the client organize his/her day and manage his/her life better, as well as day care or provision of daytime activities.
4. *Activating guidance*: e.g. talking to the client to help him/her modify behaviour or learn new forms of behaviour in cases where behavioural or psychological problems exist.
5. *Treatment*: e.g. care in connection with an ailment, such as serious absent-mindedness.
6. *Accommodation*: e.g. some people are not capable of living independent lives, but require, for example, sheltered housing or continuous supervision in connection with serious absent-mindedness. In some cases, a client's care requirements may be too great to address in a home environment, making admission to an institution necessary.

Prior to 2003, the LTC benefits covered by the AWBZ scheme were defined in terms of the type of care or the type of health-care provider people were entitled to. To encourage innovation, consumer choice and an efficient substitution of LTC services, in 2003 the definition of entitlements was radically changed into seven broad functional care categories. In 2007 one of these categories – domiciliary care – was excluded from coverage and transferred to the responsibility of the municipalities under a new Social Support Act (abbreviated WMO). The remaining six functional categories of LTC services that were covered under the AWBZ scheme in 2008 are summarized in box 1.[4]

Except for the functional category 'accommodation', clients who are entitled to care have a choice of receiving it 'in kind' or in the form of a *personal care budget* (or a combination of both). The personal care budget is set at about 75 per cent of the average cost of care provided 'in kind' because this budget can be spent on informal care, which is expected to be less expensive than professional formal care.

Expansion of LTC Services and Expenditure, 1968–2005

The enactment and gradual expansion of the public long-term insurance scheme (AWBZ) paved the way for a strong growth of long-term care facilities and of public expenditure on LTC. The percentage of GDP spent on long-term services covered by AWBZ increased from 0.8 per cent in 1968 to 2.0 per cent in 1980 and further to 4.0 per cent in 2005. Part of this increase, however, is due to an expansion of AWBZ coverage.

As shown in figure 1, from 1985 to 2000 the percentage of GDP spent on LTC services that were covered by AWBZ in 2000 was more or less stable, around 3.5 per cent (in 1985, however, only 2.0 per cent was covered by

Figure 1

Percentage of GDP spent on LTC services covered by AWBZ in the current year and in
2005, from 1985 to 2005

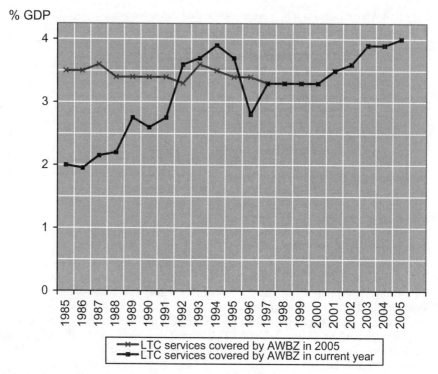

Note: From 1997 to 2005 the LTC services covered by AWBZ were the same as in 2005, so
the two lines overlap. The bubble in the black line from 1992 to 1995 is caused by a temporary inclusion of outpatient drugs into the AWBZ benefits package.
Sources: Ministry of Health (2004); Eggink *et al.* (2008).

AWBZ and 1.5 per cent was financed in other ways). Hence, taking into
account the expansion of AWBZ coverage, the expenditure on LTC services
as a percentage of GDP has been quite constant over a considerable period of
time. This is remarkable given the ageing of the population (albeit fairly
moderate during that period) and the susceptibility of LTC to Baumol's cost
disease due to the limited scope for productivity gains in the provision of care
(Oliviera Martins and Maisonneuve 2006). Despite the introduction of new
technologies in the area of healthy ageing, the quality of many LTC services
is likely to remain highly dependent on the input of labour. Therefore, the
scope of substituting capital for labour is limited.[5]

The main reason for the limited growth of public spending on LTC has
been the implementation of cost-containment policies. Already in the 1970s
the entry and capacity of new LTC institutions was strictly regulated. For

building and major investments in facilities a licence from the government was required, and only if investments were judged to be of sufficient priority was such a licence granted. Particularly important, however, was the introduction in 1984 of a system of global budgeting for all inpatient long-term health services. In addition, especially during the 1980s the government successfully mitigated the wages of nursing personnel. In the 1990s, prompted by an economic recession, the budgetary controls were expanded to include also home health care and other outpatient LTC services.

The persistent rationing of supply, postponement of investments and budgetary controls resulted in growing waiting lists and a general perception of a deterioration of quality, particularly compared to the general increase in standard of living and the rising expectations about the quality of care people would like to receive in old age. In 1999 the long waiting lists for home health care were successfully challenged in court. The court ruled that public LTC insurance entitled people to timely access to home health care, and that budgetary considerations were no valid reason for withholding care. In fact, the court decision implied that a too stringent rationing of health services was not compatible with the 'right to care' that was guaranteed by the social insurance legislation (AWBZ).

Urged on by the court decision and the mounting public and political pressure to improve access and quality of LTC services, in 2000 the government decided to lift the budgetary controls and to reimburse all extra production necessary to reduce waiting lists. Indeed, from 2000 to 2003 waiting lists were substantially reduced: for home health care by 64 per cent, for nursing homes by 39 per cent and for elderly homes by 23 per cent (Van Gameren 2005). As a consequence, during that period the expenditure on long-term care rapidly increased to more than 10 per cent per year (see figure 2), resulting in an increase from 3.5 to 4.0 per cent in the share of GDP spent on LTC (see figure 1).

During the period 1985–2005 the average annual growth of real expenditure on long-term care services covered by AWBZ was 3.3 per cent, whereas the average annual increase of GDP was about 2.7 per cent. The average difference of 0.6 per cent, however, is completely caused by the high cost inflation during the short period from 2000 to 2003. As shown in figure 3, the largest share of expenditure growth can be explained by an increase in relative prices (2.0 per cent) while about 1.3 per cent can be attributed to an increase in production.[6]

From figure 3 it can be concluded that for four of the five major categories of long-term care services the annual cost growth was about 4 per cent, which is well above the annual increase of GDP. This relatively high cost increase is largely compensated, however, by a relatively low cost increase of residential elderly care (on average about 1.3 per cent per year). This is caused by a decrease in production (on average −0.7 per cent per year) due to reductions in the capacity of elderly homes and a substitution towards home health care. As a result, the annual production growth in home health care is the largest among the five categories of LTC services (on average about 2.5 per cent per year). Clearly, this reflects the trend that elderly people are treated at home for a longer period.

Figure 2

Annual growth of LTC expenditures financed by public insurance (AWBZ)

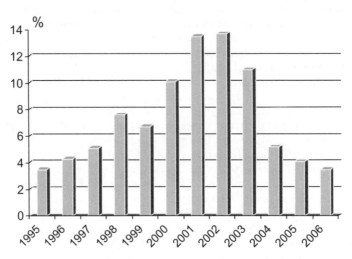

Source: IBO-werkgroep AWBZ (2006: 42).

As shown in figure 4, labour productivity for all LTC services decreased by 0.3 per cent over the entire 1985–2005 period, contributing slightly to the overall price increase. This corroborates the supposition that Baumol's cost disease is particularly relevant for LTC services (Oliviera Martins and Maisonneuve 2006). Contrary to the general trend, labour productivity in home health care increased by on average 0.7 per cent per year during the same period. The increase in labour productivity in home health care has been particularly pronounced since 1995 and is attributed to a tightening of the budgets for home health care agencies, resulting in a relative decline in administrative and managerial personnel and the introduction of benchmarking and time management to increase the efficiency of production (Eggink *et al.* 2008).

Looking at the development of long-term care expenditure in the period 1985–2000, supply regulation and budgetary restrictions were clearly quite effective in containing cost. The downside of the prolonged rationing policies, however, was increasing waiting lists, resulting in a growing public discontent and incompatibility with the legally established entitlements to LTC services. For this reason, in 2000 a continuation of the prevailing cost containment strategy was no longer politically feasible. On the other hand, the radical change towards an open-ended reimbursement policy proved to be no solution either, since the resulting excessive cost inflation – without accompanying incentives for efficiency – was not sustainable. Already in 2004 the government tried to regain control over LTC expenditure by concluding agreements with the interest associations of LTC providers to limit the growth of expenditure and to increase productivity. In addition, particu-

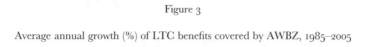

Figure 3

Average annual growth (%) of LTC benefits covered by AWBZ, 1985–2005

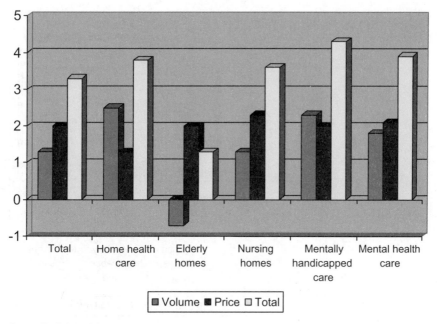

Source: Eggink *et al.* (2008).

larly for home health services, co-payments were increased. In 2005, the government reinstated budgetary controls by imposing regional budgets for each of the 32 regions, based on the past expenditure on LTC in that region. Regional care offices were made responsible for the allocation of these budgets and had to negotiate with regional providers about prices and maximum output levels. By reintroducing tight budget constraints, the government runs the risk that waiting lists will increase, which could again generate a conflict with the existing legal entitlement to LTC. In contrast to the late 1990s, however, there is an important safety valve: the personal care budget. Since personal care budgets do not fall under the scope of the regional budget constraints, LTC providers can exceed their budgets if they can persuade their clients to apply for a personal budget and to use this to pay the provider. Indeed, this is one of reasons for the vast and increasing popularity of personal care budgets.

Personal Care Budgets and Informal Care

Personal care budgets were introduced in 1995 as a small-scale experiment to provide consumers with the option to buy and organize their own home

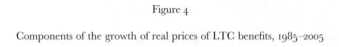

Figure 4

Components of the growth of real prices of LTC benefits, 1985–2005

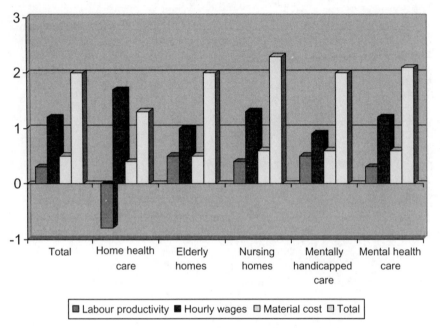

Legend: ▨ Labour productivity ■ Hourly wages ☐ Material cost ☐ Total

Source: Eggink *et al.* (2008).

health services instead of using 'in kind' services contracted by the regional care offices (Van den Berg and Hassink 2008). Since 1995 the personal care budget scheme has been significantly expanded both in scope and expenditure. As of 2008 personal care budgets comprise about 7 per cent of long-term care expenditure covered by AWBZ and are used by more than 10 per cent of LTC users. Table 3 provides some key figures about personal budgets in 2005.

There were several reasons that were put forward for the introduction of personal care budgets (Hessing-Wagner 1990). First, such budgets were considered as a means to empower consumers and to motivate providers to better meet consumer preferences. During the 1990s LTC providers were increasingly criticized for not being able to deliver the right services at the right time. Moreover, the new generation of LTC users had higher expectations and was supposed to be better able to express its preferences for LTC. By the option to choose a personal budget instead of contracted LTC services, people would be able to arrange care according to their own preferences.

A second reason for introducing personal care budgets was to encourage the use and provision of informal care as a cheap alternative to professional formal care. Informal care is a crucial part of long-term care all over the world. In the Netherlands, however, informal care plays a relatively minor role, which is partly due to the relatively generous coverage of professional formal LTC services.

Using 2004 data from the Survey of Health Ageing and Retirement in Europe (SHARE) Albertini *et al.* (2007) show that within Europe the annual amount of informal care per caregiver is lowest in the Netherlands, Denmark, France and Sweden (around 300 hours) and highest in Italy (almost 1,500 hours). Also using SHARE data, Bolin *et al.* (2008) show that the mean hours of received informal care by single-living elderly per year in the Netherlands is among the lowest within Europe (approximately 50 hours), while in Greece, Italy and Spain the single-living elderly receive the most informal care (over 200 hours). Conditional upon receiving informal care, the amount of care received by the single Dutch elderly is also among the lowest in Europe (about 130 hours per year).

In terms of professional home care use, the opposite pattern seems to hold. Bolin *et al.* (2008) show that the Netherlands (together with Denmark and France) belongs to the European top of professional home care use. Of single-living Dutch elderly, approximately 25 per cent use professional home care, while the proportion is the smallest in Italy (6 per cent).

Although the share of informal care in the Netherlands is lower than in most other European countries, still the majority of home care is provided by

Table 3

Key figures of personal care budget in 2005

Number of budget-holders: 77,883		
Age distribution (years)	18–55	32.5%
	56–65	12.6%
	66–75	14.3%
	76–80	8.7%
Type of health problem	Somatic	67%
	Psychogeriatric	1%
	Psychiatric	14%
	Physical handicap	14%
	Mental handicap	11%
	Sensory handicap	1%
Net budget amount (euros)*	<2,500	27.7%
	2500–5000	24.9%
	5000–25,000	30.5%
	>25,000	16.9%
Proportion of budget spent on informal care	Resident providers	21%
	Non-resident providers	17%

*Net of co-payments by budget-holder. The average gross personal care budget was about €14,000, of which about €1,000 was paid by the budget-holder out-of-pocket.
Source: Ministry of Health (2006).

informal caregivers. Table 4 shows that in the Netherlands the amount of home care used in 2001 was just around 15 per cent of the total amount of informal care provided. Nevertheless, table 4 also shows the enormous growth of professional home care use (especially skilled housework) during the relatively short period 2000–3.

The rapid expansion of personal care budgets was an effective way to encourage the provision of informal care. In 2005, some 38 per cent of personal care budgets were spent on informal care, while two-thirds of budget-holders use the budget for paying informal caregivers (Ramakers and Van den Wijngaart 2005). Next to personal care budgets, the role of informal care was also increased by restricting the possibilities for substituting professional for informal care. Initially, using informal care was considered to be people's voluntary choice. Even people having a social network with potential informal caregivers could always apply to get professional care that was covered by the AWBZ. In practice, however, the needs assessment agencies increasingly took into account the amount of informal care a client already received in order to determine the amount of professional care the client could legally claim (Jörg et al. 2002). Since 2003, this practice has been formalized, and strict protocols were developed regarding needs assessments, taking into account the potential amount of informal care the care recipient's social network could provide.

Another way to encourage the provision of informal care was to support informal caregivers. To prevent these caregivers getting health problems themselves, needs assessment agencies were permitted to refer caregivers to regional support centres. The support centres developed all kinds of respite care programmes, such as day care, short stays in nursing homes, holidays, and informational support (see e.g. Koopmanschap et al. 2004; Van Exel et al. 2006).

Evaluative studies point out that, as intended, personal care budgets induced a substitution of informal for professional care, and were valued by many clients as an effective means to purchase and organize care that better meets their preferences than regular care contracted by regional care offices (Ramakers et al. 2007). However, personal care budgets also had several unintended negative effects. First, they induced a substitution of paid for unpaid informal care. Informal care by relatives, neighbours and friends that previously was often provided for free, was becoming increasingly paid for. A study among informal caregivers pointed out that 76 per cent of the caregivers would be willing to provide the same care without receiving payment, although 78 per cent indicated that getting paid nevertheless was important to them (Ramakers and Van den Wijngaart 2005). In addition, an increasing number of brokers became active, who in return for a fee offered to assist people in applying for a personal care budget. Van den Berg and Schut (2003) calculated that a substitution of paid for unpaid informal care from the personal care budget could result in an increase of AWBZ costs of approximately €4 billion per year (about 20 per cent of total AWBZ expenditure).[7] Counteracting the substitution of paid for unpaid informal care was another reason for implementing the above-mentioned strict needs assessment protocols that explicitly take into account the amount of informal care that the recipient's social network could

Table 4

Hours of professional and informal home care provided per year, 2000–3 (000)

	2000		2001		2002		2003	
	Hours (000)	Share (%)	Hours (000)	Share (%)	Hours (000)	Share (%)	Hours (000)	Share (%)
Home care								
Unskilled housework	13,220	22.4	13,512	21.3	12,545	18.1	12,529	16.6
Skilled housework	16,425	27.9	18,911	29.9	22,653	32.6	26,237	34.7
Total housework	29,645	–	32,423	–	35,198	–	38,766	–
Personal care[a]	23,029	39.1	23,877	37.7	25,733	37.0	27,541	36.5
Nursing[b]	6,259	10.6	7,028	11.1	8,536	12.3	9,249	12.2
Total home care	58,933	100	63,328	100	69,467	100	75,556	100
Informal care								
All tasks[c]			375,000					

[a]Including specialized personal care.
[b]Including specialized nursing.
[c]Calculated assuming that informal caregivers provide on average 5 hours care per day, for four days per week for 25 weeks per year.
Source: Van den Berg (2004).

provide. According to the protocols, needs were not only based on health status or functional impairments but also on the availability of 'usual care'. For instance, the care partners provide to each other during at least three months is defined as usual care. Hence, the magnitude of the personal care budget became explicitly dependent on the social network of the beneficiary. Nevertheless, it is unclear to what extent people still can use personal care budgets for replacing unpaid with paid informal care. Especially, the fast-increasing number of personal care budgets for the assistance of young people with psychiatric disorders has been attributed to the substitution of paid for unpaid informal care provided by their parents.

A second drawback was that personal budgets were increasingly used by home health care agencies to escape the imposed budget constraints. As a consequence also, people who did not want to purchase and arrange care for themselves were more or less forced to do so in order to be able to keep the same home care provider.

It is difficult to assess to what extent personal care budgets were successful in accomplishing the aims behind their introduction. The rapidly increasing number of people opting for a personal care budget suggests that for a substantial proportion of users of outpatient LTC the budgets offered better opportunities to meet consumer preferences than care in kind. The problem is, however, that there is not much empirical information about the true motives of people to opt for the personal care budget. For instance, the growing demand for personal care budgets can at least partly be explained by the motivation to evade waiting lists for traditionally financed LTC and by consumer preferences to pay formerly unpaid informal caregivers. It is also unclear to what extent personal care budgets induced an efficient substitution of informal for formal care or just an expansion of paid informal care. For instance, the increasing number of parents opting for a personal care budget to provide care for their children seems to point to a substitution of paid for unpaid informal care. Moreover, for this group of clients it is unlikely that empowerment and better consumer-directed care were the main drivers to opt for a personal budget. In contrast, it seems fair to conclude that for people with long-term disabilities, personal care budgets really provide an instrument that helps them to empower themselves and to purchase care that better meets their preferences than care in kind.

Projections of Future LTC Expenditure

Future expenditure on LTC depends on a number of factors, both demographic and non-demographic. Several projections of future LTC expenditures have been made, which are not completely comparable because they are based on different definitions of LTC and use different assumptions and methodologies.

In a study about the drivers of public LTC expenditures (primarily elderly care), Oliviera Martins and Maisonneuve (2006) explicitly model the potential determinants of future LTC expenditure to project the expected share of GDP spent on LTC in 2050 for 30 OECD countries. The main results of their projections for the Netherlands and average OECD are summarized in table 5.

Since the dependency on LTC increases sharply with age, demographic effects contribute to a substantial increase in LTC expenditures. The effects of ageing on LTC consumption might be mitigated by a 'healthy ageing' process if longevity gains are fully or partially translated in additional years of good health. Since the empirical evidence about the occurrence (and extent) of a healthy ageing process is mixed, Oliviera Martins and Maisonneuve (2006) assume that only half of the longevity gains are translated into a reduction in dependency.[8] In addition, they also estimate the effect of a full healthy ageing process (compression of disability) and a complete absence of healthy ageing (expansion of disability).

In projecting future LTC expenditures, Oliviera Martins and Maisonneuve (2006) capture the Baumol effect by assuming that unit costs rise in line with aggregate labour productivity, a proxy for wage growth of care staff. As shown in table 5, this full Baumol effect induces a steady increase in relative prices, pushing LTC expenditures to 3.7 per cent of GDP in the Netherlands and to 3.3 per cent for the OECD countries on average. In addition, the effects of potential cost containment policies were simulated assuming that governments would be able to mitigate the cost pressures associated with the Baumol effect, by stimulating productivity gains and mitigating wage increase.

Under the base scenario, Oliviera Martins and Maisonneuve (2006) assume an income elasticity of zero, since they argue that LTC can be characterized as a necessity. Although empirical evidence of income elasticities for LTC are lacking, estimated income elasticities for health care in general are all above unity at a country level (Getzen 2000). This suggests that – at least for industrialized countries – health care can be considered as a luxury. Since the substitution of professional care for informal care can be seen as a luxury that may be only publicly affordable if a country as a whole reaches a certain aggregate income level, long-term care may well be a luxury rather than a necessity. If this is true, the result of the sensitivity analysis using a unitary income elasticity may be more relevant. Table 5 shows that this implies that in 2050 an extra 0.5 per cent of GDP would be spent on LTC.

The authors also estimate the effect of an increase in dependency as a result of increasing disability rates (assumed to be 0.5 per cent per year) due to a continuation of the current trends in obesity. Finally, the authors examine the impact of an 'increased participation' scenario in which the availability of informal care is dramatically reduced by assuming that all countries converge towards a labour participation ratio in the age group of 50–64 years (which is used as a proxy for the availability of informal care) of at least 70 per cent by 2050. As shown in table 5, both an increase in dependency and an increase in labour market participation are likely to have a substantial impact on LTC expenditure in the Netherlands and other OECD countries.

Specific projections of the future cost of LTC in the Netherlands have been made by the Netherlands Institute for Social Research (SCP) and the Dutch National Bureau for Economic Research (CPB). Based on the expected growth of the number of users, the SCP study projected an annual growth of

Table 5

Projection scenarios for public LTC expenditure,* 2005–2050 (% of GDP)

| | % of GDP in 2005 | Demographic effect | Full Baumol effect | Cost containment | Sensitivity analysis (compared to cost containment scenario) | | | | |
					Unitary income elasticity	Compression of disability	Expansion of disability	Increase in dependency	Increased participation
					% of GDP in 2050				
Netherlands	1.7	2.4	3.7	2.9	3.5	2.4	3.4	4.1	3.9
Average of 30 OECD countries	1.1	2.3	3.3	2.4	2.9	1.9	2.8	3.5	3.9

*According to a narrow definition of LTC, including primarily elderly care (accounting for about 45 per cent of expenditures covered by AWBZ).
Source: Oliviera Martins and Maisonneuve (2006).

expenditure on home health care, elderly homes and nursing home care of about 1.3 per cent in constant prices for the period 2005–30 (Eggink *et al.* 2008). The projected increase in cost is higher than the projected increase in the number of users, which can be explained by the higher expected growth in the number of users of the most expensive LTC facilities (especially nursing homes).

The CPB followed another methodology to project future expenditure on LTC (SER 2008). After making the observation that expenditures on LTC are very sensitive to the type of government policy, the CPB made a distinction between two extreme scenarios. The first is based on a prolonged policy of supply and price regulation as in the period 1990–2000. Since during this period the annual growth of LTC expenditure was 0.6 per cent lower than the growth of GDP, the CPB assumes that under this scenario the same difference in growth would occur during the next decade. This would result in a decline in the proportion of GDP spent on LTC to 3.5 per cent in 2020 (using a broad definition of LTC, as in this chapter). The second scenario is based on a prolonged policy of *laissez faire*, as was prevalent from 2000 to 2006. During this period the annual rise in expenditure on LTC was about 3.8 per cent higher than the growth of GDP. Using this figure as the relevant difference under the second scenario, the resulting share of GDP spent on LTC in 2020 would be 6.4 per cent.

Since both extreme scenarios are unlikely, the 3.5 and 6.4 per cent of GDP can be perceived as lower and upper bounds on the LTC expenditure in 2020 (using a broad definition of LTC). The crucial role of health policy is in line with the observation by the OECD (2005) that the correlation across countries between LTC spending and ageing is rather weak, suggesting that the way of organizing and financing LTC plays an important role.

The overall conclusion that emerges from these projections is that the future expenditure on LTC are extremely uncertain and very sensitive to the exact growth of the number of elderly, changes in real prices of LTC (due to changes in labour productivity and the quality and intensity of care), changes in health policy, changes in labour market participation and trends in disability among the elderly.

Deficiencies of Current LTC Financing

The projections of future expenditure on long-term care make clear that a *laissez faire* policy without supply and demand constraints (as in the period 2000–3) is likely to jeopardize the sustainability of the public LTC insurance scheme. On the other hand, a return to the stringent top–down rationing policy of the 1990s has serious drawbacks and does not seem feasible either. Faced with this dilemma, the government has temporarily opted for a mixture of the two policies, half-heartedly relying on both supply constraints and arrangements to improve efficiency by increasing consumer direction and choice. For the following reasons, this inconsistent policy compromise can achieve neither cost containment nor an effective increase in efficiency.

First, the currently imposed supply constraints in the form of regional care budgets are not effective in controlling cost because they can be circumvented by opting for a personal care budget. Since personal care budgets are not included under the regional budget, the regional budget constraint is not binding. Although the government introduced a separate macro budget for personal care budgets, particularly since 2005 the demand for personal care budgets has been much larger than the available funds. Rather than denying personal care budgets, the government regularly adjusts the macro budget upwards to meet the growing demand. In 2007, for instance, the government decided four times to raise the budget, resulting in a total annual budget increase of 35 per cent (Ministry of Health 2007).

Second, the regional budget mechanism punishes providers who do a good job and consequently attract more clients than the target number on which their budget is based. If these presumably efficient providers cannot effectively motivate their clients to apply for a personal care budget, they have to refuse clients or run a deficit.

Third, regional care offices do not have an incentive to allocate the regional budget to the most efficient providers because they have a regional monopoly and are not at risk for the cost of care. Since LTC users cannot choose another regional care office, these offices have no incentive to allocate budgets to providers that best meet consumer preferences. Again, consumers may opt for a personal care budget (except for inpatient care), but this is not likely to discipline the behaviour of the regional offices because they do not benefit from having more customers. Moreover, since regional offices get a fixed budget for administrative cost, they have a financial incentive to negotiate with a limited number of large providers in order to minimize the cost of contracting. For the same reason, regional care offices have no incentive to take action against over-lenient needs assessment procedures.

Finally, the definition of entitlements in terms of six functional categories (see box 1) has proven to be too imprecise to provide a firm basis for uniform and unambiguous needs assessment. In particular, the number of clients that were assessed to be in need of 'supportive guidance' increased dramatically, by 37 per cent from 2005 to 2007 (Ministry of Health 2008).

Proposals to Reform LTC Financing

In view of the serious deficiencies of the current system of LTC financing, the government asked a number of advisory and supervisory bodies[9] to draft proposals for reforming the system of LTC financing in order to guarantee a sustainable, efficient and consumer-directed provision of LTC.

This resulted in five different advisory reports, which were not all equivocal. Reports by the Council on Health Insurance (CVZ) and the Council of Public Health and Care (RVZ) recommended the complete abolition of the separate public long-term insurance scheme. Most of the benefits covered by AWBZ had to be included into the new national Health Insurance Act for curative health services (abbreviated ZVW) and the remaining benefits (related to social support and participation) into the new Social Support Act (abbreviated WMO). The main line of reasoning was that the new health insurance scheme for curative services – based on the model of managed competition (Van de Ven and Schut 2008) – would provide much stronger incentives for efficiency and meeting consumer preferences than the AWBZ. Moreover, integrating curative and long-term care into a single scheme would also provide incentives and possibilities for a better coordination of care for people with chronic diseases. Next, the original reasons for a separate public insurance scheme (see the section on background, above) were no longer valid, since the mandatory insurance scheme for curative services was extended to the entire population in 2006. Finally, the 2007 Social Support Act (WMO) provided an integrated legal framework for social and community support under the responsibility of municipalities, so the transfer of social care benefits from the AWBZ to the WMO would also enhance a better coordination of social care and welfare assistance.

The radical proposals to abolish the AWBZ scheme, however, also had serious potential shortcomings. Most importantly, it is questionable whether the model of managed competition underlying the new health insurance scheme for curative services is adequate for the provision and financing of long-term care (Van de Ven and Schut 1994). A key element of the managed competition model, which makes it possible to guarantee universal access in a competitive health insurance market, is an adequate system of risk adjustment (Van de Ven and Schut 2008). At present, there are no appropriate risk adjusters available for LTC and it is even unclear whether adequate risk adjustment is feasible for many of these services (IBO-werkgroep AWBZ 2006). Given the typically high level of expenditure per LTC user and the intertemporal nature of the risk, imperfect risk adjustment for these types of services may result in unfair competition among insurers and huge incentives for risk selection if insurers are obliged to charge community-rated premiums (as is the case under the 2006 Health Insurance Act). Another reason why the managed competition model may not be appropriate for LTC services is that for many of these services consumers are not able or willing to make an informed choice among health insurers that contract these services. There is substantial empirical evidence that the propensity to switch health plans substantially declines with age and the presence of health problems (Strombom et al. 2002; Schut et al. 2003; Buchmueller 2006). For LTC services for which the number of critical buyers is too small, competition may result in a deterioration of quality, since competitive health insurers may have an incentive to reduce quality in order to reduce cost if this does not result in a significant loss of market share (Van de Ven and Schut 1994). Finally, the experience with both the new Health Insurance Act and the new Social Support Act is limited and it is unclear whether health insurers and municipalities are willing and able to perform as prudent purchasers of health and social services. Therefore, a major expansion of the scope of the responsibilities of health insurers and municipalities would be premature.

In view of these shortcomings, other advisory reports proposed to maintain a separate insurance scheme for several categories of LTC, at least including care for the mentally handicapped. Among these reports, the proposal by the Social and Economic Council was the latest and the most important (SER 2008). The SER proposed to reform the AWBZ along the following main lines:

1. A much more precise and unambiguous delineation and definition of entitlements.
2. An improvement of the needs assessment by developing uniform protocols, benchmarking and a permanent supervision of the assessment bodies.
3. A reduction of coverage by transferring short-term rehabilitation services to the health insurance scheme for curative health services (Health Insurance Act) and by bringing the provision of social care under the responsibility of the municipalities (Social Support Act).
4. A far-reaching separation of the financing of accommodation and care, implying that accommodation would no longer be reimbursed by public insurance; a subsidy scheme for lower-income groups to pay for the cost of accommodation; the separation of care and accommodation should lead to innovative combinations of accommodation, care, welfare and participation.
5. A replacement of provider-based budgeting by client-based budgeting. Rather than clients having to follow the money – as in the current provider-based budgeting system – the money should follow the client. Clients would have the option to choose a personal care budget (as in the current system) and arrange all care by themselves, or to choose among providers contracted by individual health insurers (that would have to replace regional care offices in 2012). Providers can increase revenues if they are able to attract more clients by offering better service (for a fixed budget per client). The client-based budgets should be based on the categorization of clients in 'care-severity packages' (abbreviated ZZPs) by the needs assessment bodies. A 'care-severity package' describes the type and amount of care needed by the client. For each 'care-severity package' a budget will be calculated.

In June 2008 the government declared its endorsement of the main lines of the SER proposal and announced the first steps to implement its recommendations, including a more precise demarcation of entitlements and an exclusion of recovery and social support from coverage by 2009 (Ministry of Health 2008). In a subsequent policy letter by mid-2009, the reform plans were further elaborated (Ministry of Health 2009). In this letter the government stated its aim of abolishing the regional care offices in 2012 and instead making individual health insurers responsible for the purchasing and contracting of LTC services on behalf of their insured (next to maintaining the option for clients to choose a personal care budget or voucher and to purchase care by themselves). However, this decision is made contingent on the possibility of making health insurers financially accountable for the LTC expenses of their insured and on the feasibility of an adequate system of client-based budgeting.

Towards Sustainable LTC Financing?

Whether the proposed reform will lead to sustainable financing and more consumer-directed provision of long-term care services crucially depends on the ability to develop a clear-cut definition of entitlements, to improve the accuracy of needs assessment,[10] and to develop appropriate 'care-severity packages' as a solid basis for client-based budgeting. The feasibility of these three requirements is highly uncertain. In particular, client-based budgeting may turn out to be complicated. In 2008, 'care-severity packages' (ZZPs) have been developed for inpatient care, which from 2009 to 2011 will be phased in to determine the budgets for inpatient care LTC facilities (i.e. nursing homes, elderly homes, institutions for the mentally and physically handicapped and mental care institutions). The experience with these care-severity packages for financing inpatient care may make clear whether they can provide a firm basis for client-based financing. A key question will be whether the predictable cost variation per care package will be small enough to avoid problems of cream-skimming and misallocation of funds.[11] The first experiences with the introduction of client-based budgeting for inpatient LTC were evaluated by the Dutch Healthcare Authority (NZa 2009). The NZa reported that it received signals from both health-care providers and regional care offices of strategic upcoding (classifying clients in higher ZZPs than indicated) and risk selection (avoiding patients that are unprofitable given the ZZP capitation payment). The main reason put forward for such behaviour was that for several ZZPs or for several patients classified within a certain ZZP, capitation payments were insufficient to cover the costs. Based on the limited available data, the NZa could not determine whether upcoding and risk selection indeed occurred, but it announced its intention to monitor this type of behaviour and to examine the accuracy of ZZP payments.

An important, yet unanswered question is how future client-based budgets should be determined: should they be based on the average cost of all providers that offer the care package? Given the increasing pressure to contain public expenditure on LTC services, the most likely outcome may be that the client-based budgets will be derived from the regional budgets (or a national budget) set by the government, using the care-severity packages as relative weights for determining the (regional) level of the client-based budget for each care package.[12] The way of determining the budget will be closely related to another still unanswered question, namely for which party the client-based budget should be binding. In other words, if the actual cost of providing a care package differs from the client-based budget, then who should bear the additional costs or keep the residual: the client, the provider, or the insurer contracting the provider? At present, providers receive the full ZZP capitation payments for each client they serve and neither clients nor regional care offices bear financial risk (except for the income-related co-payments clients have to pay). However, if risk-bearing health insurers replace regional care offices by 2012, it is conceivable that ZZP capitation payments will be given to the insurers, which subsequently have to negotiate prices per ZZP with various LTC providers.

In theory, the Dutch proposed reforms involve appropriate incentives to improve the sustainability of the comprehensive LTC insurance scheme. As argued, in practice the success of the reforms will depend heavily on the way entitlements are defined, an improvement of the accuracy of needs assessment and the feasibility of determining appropriate client-based budgets. For adequate client-based budgeting it is crucial that the care-severity packages that are currently being developed are relatively homogeneous in terms of predicted costs as substantial variation involves clear incentives for upcoding and risk selection.

Although the proposed reform offers a promising perspective to combine a sustainable and universally accessible LTC financing with a consumer-directed provision of care, a number of complicated issues have to be resolved. The Dutch experiences in implementing the reform may therefore provide important lessons for countries with a public insurance scheme for long-term care – e.g. Japan and Germany – that also struggle with the question of how to guarantee a sustainable, universally accessible and high-quality system of long-term care (Ikegami 2007; see also Rothgang, this volume). In addition, it may also provide important lessons for countries considering the introduction of a system of social insurance for long-term care (see Barr, this volume).

Acknowledgements

A previous draft of this chapter was presented at the 7th World Congress of the international Health Economics Association (iHEA) in Beijing and at the International Conference on the Policies and Regulations of Health and Long-term Care Costs of the Elderly in Tokyo. Part of this research has been supported by a research grant to Hitotsubashi University from the Ministry of Education of Japan (grant number 18002001).

Notes

1. There are several reasons why private markets fail to provide adequate insurance for LTC. The absence of private LTC insurance has been explained (e.g. Cutler 1996; Brown and Finkelstein 2007) by the nature of intertemporal risk, by supply-side market failure (resulting from high transaction costs, adverse selection and imperfect competition) and by demand-side factors such as limited consumer rationality, limited foresight, and the availability of imperfect but cheaper substitutes.
2. As of 2008, this Centre for Needs Assessment (CIZ) has one main office, six district offices and 30 local offices.
3. Following the recently proposed typology by Ariizumi (2008), the Dutch public insurance system can be characterized as a health-based rather than a means-tested programme.
4. As of 2009, two functional categories – supportive and activating guidance – are combined into a single category 'guidance'. At the same time, guidance that is aimed at social participation is excluded from coverage and brought under the scope of the Social Support Act (WMO).
5. When productivity growth in the LTC sector lags behind that in other sectors while wages grow at the same rate, relative prices of LTC vis-à-vis other goods and services in the economy will rise. In the case of a low price elasticity of demand for LTC – which is likely in the presence of public insurance – the share of LTC expenditure in GDP will also increase over time.
6. Production of LTC services is measured by the Netherlands Institute for Social Research (Eggink et al. 2008) using indicators of production (e.g. admissions, day treatments, length of stay, number of patients, etc.) weighted by the type and intensity of treatment.

7. This number was based on the assumption that a substantial proportion of informal caregivers already get paid from the personal care budget (see also Van den Berg and Hassink 2008). Their average payment is around €10 per hour. Multiplication of this average payment with the informal care hours presented in table 4 makes approximately €4 billion.
8. For the Netherlands this assumption might be an underestimation. In the Netherlands the ratio of disability-free life expectancy to life expectancy at age 65 was 79 per cent for men and 67 per cent for women in 2000 (OECD 2005). The ratio has increased since 1990, particularly for women.
9. Specifically, the Social and Economic Council (SER), the Council for Public Health and Health Care (RVZ), the Health Care Insurance Board (CVZ), the Dutch Healthcare Authority (NZa), and a governmental working group (IBO).
10. In the Japanese LTC insurance scheme, for instance, nationally uniform standardized eligibility criteria are used to determine which services the elderly are entitled to (Ikegami 2007).
11. The determination of adequate ZZP capitation payments for outpatient LTC may be more complicated because the need for outpatient care crucially depends on the availability of a social network of informal caregivers, which typically varies substantially across individuals.
12. Using national rather than regional budgets may be politically attractive because then government may avoid a socially controversial regional variation in the level of client-based budgets.

References

Albertini, M., Kohli, M. and Vogel, C. (2007), Intergenerational transfers of time and money in European families: common patterns – different regimes? *Journal of European Social Policy*, 17: 319–34.

Ariizumi, H. (2008), Effects of public long-term care insurance on consumption, medical care demand, and welfare, *Journal of Health Economics*, 27: 1423–35.

Bolin, K., Lindgren, B. and Lundborg, P. (2008), Informal and formal care among single-living elderly in Europe, *Health Economics*, 17: 393–409.

Brown, J. R. and Finkelstein, A. (2007), Why is the market for long-term care insurance so small? *Journal of Public Economics*, 91: 1967–91.

Buchmueller, T. C. (2006), Price and the health plan choice of retirees, *Journal of Health Economics*, 25, 1: 81–101.

Cutler, D. (1996), Why don't markets insure long-term risk? Unpublished working paper. Available at: www.economics.harvard.edu/faculty/cutler/files/ltc_rev.pdf.

Eggink, E., Pommer, E. and Woittiez, I. (2008), *De ontwikkeling van de AWBZ-uitgaven: een analyse van de AWBZ-uitgaven 1985–2005 en een raming van de uitgaven voor verpleging en verzorging 2005–2030* [The development of AWBZ expenditures: an analysis of AWBZ expenditures from 1985 to 2005 and a forecast of the expenditures on nursing and care for 2005–2030], The Hague: Sociaal en Cultureel Planbureau (SCP).

Getzen, T. E. (2000), Health care is an individual necessity and a national luxury: applying multilevel decision models to the analysis of health care expenditures, *Journal of Health Economics*, 19, 2: 259–70.

Hessing-Wagner, J. C. (1990), *Cliëntgebonden budget en zorg: de individualisering van geldstromen nader beschouwd* [Client-based budget and care: a closer look at the individualization of payment flows], The Hague: Sociaal en Cultureel Planbureau (SCP).

IBO-werkgroep AWBZ (2006), *Toekomst AWBZ: Eindrapportage van de werkgroep Organisatie romp AWBZ* [The future of AWBZ: final report of the working group on the organization of the core AWBZ], Interdepartementaal Beleidsonderzoek 2004–2005, no. 4, The Hague.

Ikegami, N. (2007), Rationale, design and sustainability of long-term care insurance in Japan – in retrospect, *Social Policy and Society*, 6, 3: 423–34.

Jörg, F., Boeije, H. R., Huijsman, R., De Weert, G. H. and Schrijvers, A. J. P. (2002), Objectivity in needs assessment practice: admission to a residential home, *Health and Social Care in the Community*, 10, 6: 445–56.

Koopmanschap, M. A., Van Exel, N. J. A., Van den Bos, G. A. M., Van den Berg, B. and Brouwer, W. B. F. (2004), The desire for support and respite care: preferences of Dutch informal caregivers, *Health Policy*, 68: 309–20.

Ministry of Health (2004), *Op weg naar een bestendig stelsel voor langdurige zorg en maatschappelijke ondersteuning* [On track towards a sustainable system for long-term care and social support], Letter to parliament, DVVO-U-2475093, The Hague.

Ministry of Health (2006), Fact sheet personal budget AWBZ. Available at: www.minvws.nl/en/folders/zzoude_directies/dvvo/2005/fact-sheet-personal-budget-awbz.asp.

Ministry of Health (2007), *Pgb in perspectief* [Personal care budget in perspective], Letter to parliament, DLZ/ZI-U-2811809 (9 November), The Hague.

Ministry of Health (2008), *Zeker van zorg, nu en straks* [Assured care, now and later], Letter to parliament, DLZ/KZ-2856771 (13 June), The Hague.

Ministry of Health (2009), *Nadere uitwerking toekomst van de AWBZ* [Further details on the future of AWBZ], Letter to parliament, DLZ/CB-U-2912189 (12 June), The Hague.

NZa (2009), *Voortgangsrapportage Invoering ZZP's: Rapportage over de periode 1 januari 2009–30 juni 2009* [Proceedings on the implementation of ZZPs: report on the period 1 January 2009–30 June 2009], Utrecht: Dutch Healthcare Authority (NZa).

OECD (2005), *Long-term Care for Older People*, Paris: OECD.

Oliviera Martins, J. and Maisonneuve, C. de la (2006), The drivers of public expenditure on health and long-term care: an integrated approach, *OECD Economic Studies*, 43, 2: 115–54.

Ramakers, C. and Van den Wijngaart, M. (2005), *Persoonsgebonden budget en mantelzorg: Onderzoek naar de aard en de omvang van betaalde en onbetaalde mantelzorg* [Personal care budget and informal care: inquiry into the nature and extent of paid and unpaid informal care], Nijmegen: ITS/Radboud University.

Ramakers, C., Graauw, K. de, Sombekke, E., Vierke, H., Doesborgh, J., and Wolderingh, C. (2007), *Evaluatie persoongebonden budget nieuwe stijl 2005–2006* [Evaluation of the new version of the personal budget 2005–2006], Nijmegen: ITS/Radboud University.

Schut, F. T., Greß, S. and Wasem, J. (2003), Consumer price sensitivity and social health insurer choice in Germany and the Netherlands, *International Journal of Health Care Finance and Economics*, 3: 117–38.

SER (2008), *Langdurige zorg verzekerd: over de toekomst van de AWBZ* [Long-term care assured: about the future of the AWBZ], Publicatienummer 3, The Hague: Social and Economic Council (SER).

Strombom, B. A., Buchmueller, T. C. and Feldstein, P. J. (2002), Switching costs, price sensitivity and health plan choice, *Journal of Health Economics*, 21: 89–116.

Van den Berg, B. (2004), Dragen de sterkste schouders de zwaarste lasten? Een discussie over de positie van mantelzorgers ten opzichte van de AWBZ-zorg [Do the strongest shoulders carry the heaviest burden? A discussion about the position of informal caregivers in relation to AWBZ care], *Tijdschrift voor Politieke Ekonomie*, 26: 24–37.

Van den Berg, B. and Hassink, W. H. J. (2008), Cash benefits in long-term home care, *Health Policy*, 88: 209–21.

Van den Berg, B., and Schut, F. T. (2003), Het einde van gratis mantelzorg? [The end of free informal care?], *Economisch Statistische Berichten*, 88, 4413: 420–2.

Van de Ven, W. P. M. M. and Schut, F. T. (1994), Should catastrophic risks be included in a regulated competitive health insurance market? *Social Science and Medicine*, 39, 10: 1459–72.

Van de Ven, W. P. M. M. and Schut, F. T. (2008), Universal mandatory health insurance in the Netherlands: a model for the United States? *Health Affairs*, 27, 3: 771–81.

Van Exel, N. J. A., Morée, M., Koopmanschap, M. A., Schreuder Goedheijt, T. and Brouwer, W. B. F. (2006), Respite care: an explorative study of demand and use in Dutch informal caregivers, *Health Policy*, 78: 194–208.

Van Gameren, E. (2005), *Regionale verschillen in de wachtlijsten verpleging en verzorging: Een empirisch onderzoek naar verklarende factoren* [Regional variation in waiting lists for nursing and care: an empirical investigation of explanatory factors], Werkdocument 119, The Hague: Sociaal en Cultureel Planbureau (SCP).

5

Social Insurance for Long-term Care: An Evaluation of the German Model

Heinz Rothgang

Introduction

Although the need for long-term care (LTC) is not new, for many decades welfare states did not address it as a specific social risk. Apart from the Nordic countries, where more universalistic approaches began in the 1940s, in most OECD countries LTC was widely understood or even defined as a family responsibility with social assistance-oriented public support (Österle and Rothgang 2010). EC Regulation 1408/71 on the coordination of social security in the European Union, for example, had no section on LTC. Only in the new coordination regulation 883/2004, not yet applicable, is long-term care explicitly mentioned. From the 1980s and 1990s, the awareness of LTC and the need to ensure more systematic coverage has started to increase in OECD countries.[1] States have implemented novel, or broadened earlier, schemes. Others are currently considering more comprehensive long-term care programmes (cf. Pavolini and Ranci 2008).

For the future, changes in the socio-economic context and in the understanding of individual, family and public responsibility will have major implications for traditional care arrangements, while care policies themselves will feed back into these perceptions. Also, the need for long-term care will further increase because of demographic trends. The relevance of LTC will grow as the number of elderly citizens increases dramatically, in absolute numbers but also in relation to people younger than 65 years. This is the result of the baby boom generation approaching retirement, but also of falling mortality rates, resulting in an increase in life expectancy of 2.5 years per decade in the EU (Com (2008) 725: 5) and low fertility rates (OECD 2007: 11). The OECD estimates that by 2030 on average 20 per cent of the population will be aged 65 years and older in OECD countries and this share will rise to 25.2 per cent by 2050. Compared to 13.8 per cent in 2005, this is an 83 per cent rise. More dramatically, the share of people aged 85 and older will grow the fastest and double from 1.5 per cent in 2005 to 3 per cent in 2030. This share will rise to 5.2 per cent by 2050, representing a 242 per cent growth when compared with the figures for 2005. As the 'oldest old' face the most severe disabilities and have therefore the greatest demand for long-term care (OECD 2007: 11–14), the growth in numbers in this group is of the highest relevance for predicting the future number of dependent people.[2] As recent data show for Germany, even today every second person depends on LTC at some point in life (Rothgang *et al.* 2008), and those who survive until the age of 60 may expect 1.3 years (men) and 2.7 years (women) on average spent in need of LTC (Rothgang *et al.* 2009).[3] Therefore, provision for this has rightfully become a major concern of modern welfare states.

So, how should welfare states cope with the need for long-term care? How should LTC be financed, provided and regulated? With respect to *financing*, different mixes between public – taxes and social insurance contributions – and private sources – savings and voluntary insurance – are feasible. Concerning *service provision*, the role of formal and informal care is of the highest relevance, while *regulation* has to deal with the (legal) norms governing the relation between funding agencies, providers of formal care and people in need of LTC and their families.

This chapter analyses the German case in order also to draw some general lessons for the organization of long-term care in other countries. The next section therefore describes the system as well as current financing and service provision patterns. After that, the achievements and weaknesses of the system are discussed. This is done by analysing the 2008 reform and the future challenges and perspectives after the reform, while the final section covers lessons that can be learned from the German experience.

Long-term Care Insurance in Germany

Until the introduction of Long-term Care Insurance (LTCI) in 1994, there was no comprehensive public system for financing long-term care in Germany. When using formal care services, dependent people (and their families) had to pay out of pocket, with only means-tested social assistance as the last resort for those who had exhausted their assets and could not otherwise afford the necessary formal care.[4] The Long-term Care Act of 1994 then changed the institutional setting fundamentally.

The institutional setting after the Long-term Care Act

Coverage. The LTCI Act of 1994 established Social Long-Term Care Insurance and mandatory private long-term care insurance, which together cover almost the whole population. Members of Statutory Health Insurance became members of the Social LTCI scheme, and those who have private health insurance were obliged to buy private (mandatory) LTCI. Since all insurance benefits are capped, private co-payments remain important, and means-tested social assistance still plays a vital role, particularly in nursing home care, where about one-third of all residents still receive social assistance.[5]

Entitlement. In contrast to, for example, the Japanese Long-term Care Insurance, in Germany entitlement is independent of the age of the dependent person. However, more than 80 per cent of all beneficiaries are aged 65 years

79

or older and more than 55 per cent are at least 80 years old.[6] In legal terms, the 'need for long-term care' (or 'dependency') refers to those people who need help with at least two basic activities of daily living (ADLs) and one additional instrumental activity of daily living (iADL) for an expected period of at least six months. Three *levels of dependency* are distinguished depending on how often assistance is needed and how long it takes a non-professional caregiver to help the dependent person (see table 1). The Medical Review Board (*Medizinischer Dienst der Krankenversicherung*, or MDK) performs the assessment for members of social LTC, while Medicproof, a private company, carries out this task for private LTCI.

Benefits. LTCI benefits are set by law. Beneficiaries may choose between home care, day and night care, and nursing home care. In home care there is choice between in-kind benefits for community care and cash benefits. Cash benefits are given directly to the dependent person, who can choose to pass the cash on to a family caregiver. The use of cash benefits is at the beneficiary's discretion – given that proper caregiving is guaranteed – and not up to care managers, care agencies or LTCI funds. Community care is provided by both non-profit and for-profit providers. Up to the benefit caps (see table 2), their bills are covered by LTCI funds. Cash and in-kind benefits may be combined; i.e. if only x per cent of claims for in-kind benefits are realized, $100 - x$ per cent of the cash benefits claims are still available.

Table 2 shows the legally fixed amounts for the most important types of benefits. As the table shows, in-kind benefits for home care are about twice as high as cash benefits. In levels I and II, benefits for nursing home care are higher than for home care. Only in level III are benefits for all types of formal care the same.

If a family caregiver is on vacation, LTCI will cover the expense of a professional caregiver for a period of up to four weeks, and a ceiling of

Table 1

Definition of dependency

	Level I	Level II	Level III
Need of care with basic ADLs	At least once a day with at least two ADLs	At least thrice a day at different times of the day	Help must be available around the clock
Need of care with instrumental ADLs	More than once a week	More than once a week	More than once a week
Required time for help in total	At least 1.5 hours a day, with at least 0.75 hours for ADLs	At least 3 hours a day with at least 2 hours for ADLs	At least 5 hours a day with at least 4 hours for ADLs

Source: §15 Social Code Book (Sozialgesetzbuch XI, SGB XI).

Table 2

Amount of LTCI benefits (major types of benefits), 2009

Level	Home care		Day and night care	Nursing home care
	Cash benefits	In-kind benefits	In-kind benefits	In-kind benefits
I (moderate)	215	420	420	1,023
II (severe)	420	980	980	1,279
III (severest)	675	1,470	1,470	1,470
Special cases		1,918		1,750

Note: Sums are given as euros per month.
Source: §§36–45 Social Code Book XI.

€1,470. This is a benefit in its own right but is weighted against other claims for home care. Since 2008 the utilization of day and night care is only weighted partly against in-kind and cash benefits. There is also a small grant for special aids, and the insurance funds offer courses for non-professional caregivers. LTCI funds pay the pension contributions of informal caregivers,[7] who are also covered by accident insurance without having to pay contributions. Since 2002, additional benefits are granted to dependent people with considerable need for general supervision and care. This group, essentially including people with dementia, people suffering from mental diseases or the mentally disabled, is entitled to a supplementary care benefit of €460 per year. In 2008, this amount was increased to €1,000 per month, or €2,000 for severer cases.

Adjustment. As all benefits are capped or lump sums, without adjustment their purchasing power declines. Federal government may adjust benefits but is not obliged to do so. Until 2008, benefits were never adjusted, not even for inflation, while, for example, prices for nursing home care went up by 10 to 15 per cent. Consequently, the purchasing power of LTCI benefits has been declining. As part of the 2008 reform, for the first time benefits have been adjusted. Moreover, the obligation to check the need for adjustment every three years has been introduced (see below).

Providers of formal care. Formal care is provided by public, private non-profit and private for-profit providers, which serve members of social and private insurance alike. Providers must have a contract with LTCI funds, which they get whenever certain formal criteria are met. As LTCI benefits are capped, potential oversupply of providers is not regarded as a problem for the insurance scheme and is rather encouraged to increase competition.

Reimbursements. Regulation of remuneration for *formal home care* differs between the 16 federal states (*Länder*). In most of the federal states about two dozen complexes of services are defined and reimbursed. Remuneration levels are negotiated between LTCI funds and providers. In some of the federal states levels also differ between for-profit and non-profit providers. For the insured, higher prices imply a lower quantity of services that can be financed by capped LTCI benefits and thus rising opportunity costs of formal care. The demand for formal care is therefore price-sensitive, which means that providers are not always interested in higher prices. In *nursing home care*, remuneration consists of distinct rates for caring, board and lodging (so-called 'hotel costs') and investment costs. Rates for caring and hotel costs are negotiated between providers, on the one hand, and long-term care funds together with the agency responsible for social assistance, on the other. LTCI only pays a lump sum for caring. The resident pays for board and lodging as well as those care costs that exceed the LTCI benefits (table 3). Hotel costs do not include the annuities resulting from building or modernizing nursing homes. These '*investment costs*' are partly financed by the federal states. Respective regulations vary greatly. In order to help the former East Germany to 'catch up' with West Germany, from 1996 to 2003 a special programme was set up to fund an investment worth up to about €500 million a year in East Germany. The central government covered 80 per cent of this amount as long as the federal state in question provided the remaining 20 per cent share. Investment costs that are not publicly financed are passed on to the resident, or eventually to social assistance.

Co-payments. LTCI funds benefits are, in general, not sufficient to cover the costs of formal care at home or in a nursing home. As table 3 reveals, in nursing home care LTCI benefits are even insufficient to cover average daily rates for caring. Since residents have to pay for board and lodging out-of-pocket, co-payments are quite substantial, particularly as an average monthly amount of about €350 for investment costs (Augurzky *et al.* 2008: 24) is to be added.

Financing. Social LTCI financing follows the *pay-as-you-go principle*. It is financed almost exclusively by *contributions*, which are income-related but

Table 3

Average monthly rates for nursing homes, LTCI benefits, co-payments, 2007

Euros Level of care	(1) Care costs	(2) Board and lodging	(3) = (1) + (2) Daily rate (investment excluded)	(4) LTCI benefits	(5) = (1) − (4) Co-payments, care costs only	(6) = (3) − (4) Co-payment, care and hotel costs
Level I	1,307	608	1,915	1,023	284	892
Level II	1,733	608	2,341	1,279	454	1,062
Level III	2,158	608	2,766	1,432	726	1,334

Source: StBa (2009a) (1 and 2); Social Code Book XI (4).

not risk-related. Contributions are calculated as a certain share (contribution rate) of certain parts of the income ('contributory income'). In the case of those who are employed, employers and employees each pay 50 per cent of the contribution,[8] while contributions for the unemployed are paid by unemployment insurance. Since 2004, pensioners pay the whole contribution themselves. From July 1996 until June 2008 contributions were calculated as 1.7 per cent of gross earnings or accordingly retirement pensions up to an income ceiling of €3,675 per month (2009 figure), which is adjusted annually. Income from other sources such as assets or income from rent and leases is not considered in calculating contributions. The contribution rate can only be changed by an act of Parliament. In July 2008 the contribution rate was raised by 0.25 percentage points (see the section on the 2008 Reform, below). From 2004 onwards, insured people aged 23 or older who have never been parents have had to pay an *additional contribution* of 0.25 per cent of contributory income. Private mandatory LTCI is a partially funded scheme. Private insurance premiums are not income-related but risk-related. However, legally fixed premium caps prevent prohibitive premiums for the elderly and thereby introduce an element of redistribution between younger and older insurees.

Administration. Social LTCI is administered by different *LTCI funds*. They are responsible for contracts with care providers (including admission to the market), prices (for in-kind care), and cash benefits. Since the benefits, as well as the contribution rate, are identical for all funds and all expenses are financed by the sum of all contributions – irrespective of which fund is responsible – there is no competition between these funds (Jacobs 1995).

Provision of care and service utilization

Development of the number of beneficiaries. Long-term care insurance was phased in gradually. The first contributions were due in January 1995, but benefits for home care did not start being dispensed until April 1995. Nursing home care benefits only came into being in July 1996. From 1996 to 1999 the number of beneficiaries increased by more than a quarter of a million, clearly reflecting an introductory effect (figure 1). From 1999 to 2006 the number of beneficiaries increased from 1.826 million to 1.969 million, which represents an average growth rate of 1.1 per cent (geometric mean).[9] Thus, there has been no 'explosion' of the number of beneficiaries but rather slight but steady growth.[10]

A closer look reveals that from 1999 to 2007 the age-specific dependency rates have remained remarkably stable (Rothgang *et al.* 2009: 66–75). The growing number of beneficiaries is therefore almost completely due to demographic ageing alone. With respect to the levels of dependency, however, there is a clear trend: from 1999 to 2007 the share of beneficiaries in level I has increased from 40 to 54 per cent while at the same time the share of people in level II has decreased from 43 to 34 per cent and the share of beneficiaries in level III from 17 to 13 per cent.[11] This could be interpreted as a reflection of

Figure 1

Number of public LTCI beneficiaries at end of year

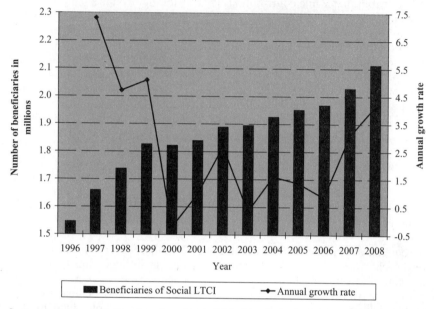

Source: Author's calculations based on data published by the Federal Ministry of Health. See: www.bmg.bund.de/cln_160/nn_1193090/SharedDocs/Downloads/DE/Statistiken/Statistiken _20 Pflege/xls-Leistungsempfaenger-am-Jahresende-nach-Altersgruppen.html.
Note: Due to statistical adjustments the numbers for 2007 and 2008 are slightly overestimated.

a compression of morbidity relating to the severity of dependency rather than to dependency as such.

Development of service utilization. There is also a gradual shift in the choice of benefits reflecting changes in the care arrangements (figure 2). The share of beneficiaries who choose cash benefits has been decreasing from more than 60 per cent in 1996 to less than 50 per cent in 2007. Though the speed of change has slowed down, the trend is still unbroken. Correspondingly, the share of dependent people in nursing home care has increased, from 23 per cent in 1996 to almost 30 per cent in 2007. Once again the amount of change is decreasing, but the trend still holds. In home care the utilization of formal care has become more important: although the share of all beneficiaries in home care decreases, the share of those who use in-kind benefits or combine formal care with cash transfers is still increasing slightly, and in 2007 for the first time exceeds the 20 per cent margin.

Though LTCI aims to strengthen home care in general and family care in particular, we rather observe a tendency towards nursing home care, and

Figure 2

Type of benefits chosen

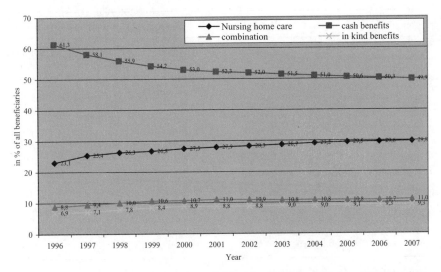

Source: Author's calculation based on data published by the Federal Ministry of Health. See: www.bmg.bund.de/cln_160/nn_1193090/SharedDocs/Downloads/DE/Pflege/Informationen/Leistungsempfaenger-nach-Leistungsarten-xls.html.

within home care towards formal care. As benefits are higher in formal care, and particularly in nursing home care, this creates an additional fiscal burden for LTCI.

Capacities of the formal sector. With respect to formal care, the LTCI Act triggered an expansion of capacity. In both nursing home care and home care, the number of providers doubled between 1992 and 1997. However, these figures should not be over-interpreted. As residential homes for the elderly were re-founded as nursing homes, and as former informal help systems (such as those organized by churches) transformed themselves into formal care providers, there are no valid time-series data showing the exact expansion of capacity immediately after the LTCI Act. Table 4, therefore, only contains – reliable – data from 1999 onwards.

From 1999 to 2007 the number of providers of home care has been growing moderately. The number of employees, on the other hand, has increased by more than one-quarter. This is due to a concentration process in the market. If only full-time employees are taken into consideration the growth rate is much lower, as the number and share of part-time jobs in this industry has increased. In nursing home care the increase in capacity is even more impressive: it has been growing by almost one-quarter, irrespective of whether the observation is based on the number of providers or the number of beds.

Table 4

The capacity of the formal care sector

	Home care			Nursing home care	
	Number of providers	Employees	Full-time employees	Number of providers	Number of beds
	Absolute numbers				
1999	10,820	183,782	56,914	8,859	645,456
2001	10,594	189,567	57,524	9,165	674,292
2003	10,619	200,897	57,510	9,743	713,195
2005	10,977	214,307	56,354	10,424	757,186
2007	11,529	236,162	62,405	11,029	799,059
	Overall growth rate (%)				
1999–2001	−2.1	3.1	1.1	3.5	4.5
2001–2003	0.2	6.0	0.0	6.3	5.8
2003–2005	3.4	6.7	−2.0	7.0	6.2
2005–2007	5.0	10.2	10.7	5.8	5.5
1999–2007	6.6	28.5	9.6	24.5	23.8

Source: StBa (2009b: 25).

Moreover, the trend still holds. Without doubt, the introduction of long-term care insurance fostered these developments.

Financing

As figure 3 demonstrates, the balance of Social LTCI deteriorated constantly from 1995 to 2004. The high surplus in 1995 was a result of granting benefits only from April onwards while collecting contributions from January onwards.[12] Even after that, it took some time for people to realize and claim the new benefits. Therefore 1996 and 1997 also show a considerable surplus. After a period of almost balanced budgets (1998–2001), results for 2002 to 2004 showed increasing deficits. This was not the result of extraordinarily high rates for expenditures. On the contrary, from 2000 – when the introductory phase was over – to 2007, the average annual growth rate (geometric mean) of nominal expenditures was just 1.4 per cent. The deficits have rather been caused by disappointing growth rates for *contributions*. From 1997 to 2004, the average annual growth rate of nominal (*sic!*) contributions was 0.8 per cent (geometric mean) – well below inflation. In 2003, contributions actually declined, and in 2004 they remained practically unchanged. Thus it is the contribution rather than the expenditure side that has caused trouble.

In December 2004, the additional contribution for those without children (see above) was introduced. Without this, the deficit for 2005 would have exceeded €1 billion. The additional revenues are permanent. For 2006, the first

Figure 3

Balance sheet of public LTCI

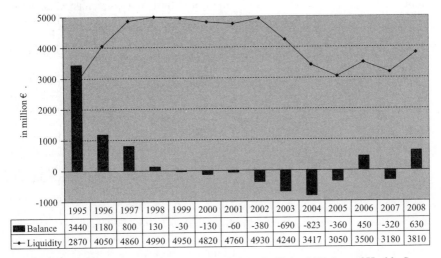

	1995	1996	1997	1998	1999	2000	2001	2002	2003	2004	2005	2006	2007	2008
■■ Balance	3440	1180	800	130	-30	-130	-60	-380	-690	-823	-360	450	-320	630
◆ Liquidity	2870	4050	4860	4990	4950	4820	4760	4930	4240	3417	3050	3500	3180	3810

Source: Author's depiction, based on data published by the Federal Ministry of Health. See:
www.bmg.bund.de/cln_100/nn_1193090/SharedDocs/Downloads/DE/Statistiken/
Statistiken_20Pflege/xls-Finanzentwicklung-der-sozialen-Pflegeversicherung-Ist-
Ergebnisse.html.

surplus in 8 years should be noted. This, however, is merely a singular effect caused by the change in due date of contributions. As a result, for employees 13 monthly contributions were collected, resulting in extra revenue of about €600 million (Rothgang and Dräther 2009: 42). Consequently, the year 2007 once again shows a deficit similar to that of 2005. In 2008, finally, a reform was enacted, which – among other things – increased the contribution rate but also some benefits (see the section on achievements and weaknesses, below).

Both developments – the moderate growth rates for expenditure and the disappointing growth rates for contributions – need to be explained. The only *moderate growth of expenditures* has been due to two major factors: First, the insurance system is based on a comparatively tight definition of dependency (see Rothgang and Comas-Herrera 2003), and entitlement for LTCI benefits is based on a rigorous assessment by the Medical Review Board. Second, all benefits are capped or are lump sums and were not adjusted from 1995 to 2008, not even for inflation. So, while the assessments have prevented any explosion of the number of beneficiaries, the benefit caps have controlled expenditure per beneficiary. Of course, there is a price to be paid for cost containment of this kind. First, the tight definition of dependency has meant that people with dementia are entitled to LTCI benefits only insofar as they need help with the activities of daily living, as the assessment does not evaluate or take into account their general need for supervision. Second, due to the benefit caps, there is still a large out-of-pocket payment, which is unusual for the traditional German social insurance system. Moreover, the number of persons in need of long-term care who depend on social assistance is still high, and much higher than had been anticipated. Finally, the fact that the benefits have never been adjusted in more than a decade has caused the purchasing power of LTCI benefits to decline. Such a strategy will eventually lead to a delegitimization of this branch of social insurance. This is why in the long run it is simply not feasible to continue cost control based on missing adjustments.

The *slow growth of contributions* is partly an effect of certain (social) policies. First, contributions are only levied on income from gainful employment and benefits derived from that (pensions, unemployment benefits), while income from other sources and income above the income ceiling is not taken into account. As a result the growth of the sum of contributory income is permanently slower than the growth of GDP. Moreover, certain changes in social law have reduced contributions either explicitly or implicitly. For example, in 2000 the federal government reduced contributions for the unemployed, which have to be financed by the unemployment insurance, because, at that time, it was beset with fiscal problems, while the LTCI had considerable assets. Similarly, the introduction of so-called mini-jobs and midi-jobs, that is, jobs paying up to €400 and €800 a month, respectively, reduced the amount of contributory income to the LTCI funds as these workers are exempt from making regular contributions. This effect is likely to become yet more noticeable as normal jobs are increasingly transformed into mini-jobs. Something similar is happening to the old-age security system. Recent legislation aims at the partial substitution of (mandatory) public schemes by (voluntary) private schemes. In the course of this legislation the federal government has introduced new opportunities for sacrificed compensation which has reduced the amount of contributory income. A general feature of social policy over the last decades has been that the problems in one branch of the insurance system have often been resolved at the expense of others. As for the existing reserve fund, the LTCI has been used as a cash cow for other branches of social security. In addition, LTCI contributions have suffered from the general trends that have affected all branches of social security, namely the reduction in the number of jobs that are subject to social insurance contributions, cyclical and structural unemployment, and low (if any) rises in wages and pensions. Thus, it is an irony of history that LTCI financing is in trouble despite successful cost-containment because of inadequate contributions, partly caused by social policy regulations aimed at solving problems in other branches of social security.

Social and private mandatory LTCI only cover part of the needs of dependent people. Table 5 therefore gives an overview of total expenditure on long-term care – excluding the value of informal care. According to the figures in the table, almost one-third of all funding is out-of-pocket, overwhelmingly spent on nursing home care. Within the public area, social long-term care covers more than 80 per cent of the expenditure, with social assistance following with 12 per cent. These figures demonstrate the major role social long-term care insurance plays in public funding, but they also highlight the considerable role of out-of-pocket funding.

Table 5

Sources of funding for long-term care

Source of funding	Million euro	% of public/ private spending	% of all spending
Public funding (total), consisting of ***	21,610	100	68.7
Public LTCI*	17,860	82.6	56.8
Private mandatory LTCI*	550	2.5	1.7
Social assistance	2,610	12.1	8.3
Welfare for war victims	590	2.7	1.9
Out-of-pocket private funding (total)** on:	9,840	100	31.3
Nursing home care	7,660		24.4
Home care	2,180		6.9
Total	*31,450*		*100*

Notes: *Cash allowances are included.
**Estimated.
***Federal states shall fund investment costs of LTC providers. Respective activities have been declining and recent figures are not published and therefore not included here.
Source: Rothgang *et al.* (2008: 88).

Achievements and Weaknesses of the System

As Barr (this volume) argues, long-term care is a suitable case for social insurance. In order to illustrate this point, it is important first to recall the *achievements* of the long-term care insurance:

- Perhaps the most important achievement is that long-term care is no longer regarded as a negligible residual risk, but as a *social risk* demanding social protection. Along with that, in § 8 Social Code Book XI long-term care has been defined as a *societal duty* (*gesamtgesellschaftliche Aufgabe*) thus giving some relief to families that are unable to take care of their elderly alone.
- Consequently, the *whole population* is covered – either in social or mandatory private LTCI – thus avoiding problems related to the uninsured. Since the insurance system is financed following the *pay-as-you-go system*, benefits could be granted immediately without a decade-long period of capital accumulation.[13]
- The introduction of the LTCI was legitimized as a means to prevent dependent elderly people with a 'standard working life' from relying on *social assistance* once they had to go to a nursing home. In fact, the respective share of residents has been diminished considerably, but still about 30 per cent of residents receive social assistance. The fiscal effect for municipalities and federal states was even more impressive: respective expenses declined to about one-third of the original value (Roth and Rothgang 2001: 295).

89

- Due to the introduction of LTCI, public expenses on LTC have immediately increased from about €8 to €20 million (Rothgang 1997: 196 ff.). This is one of the reasons for the *expansion of capacities* in the formal care sector described in the section on the provision of care and service utilization, above. Moreover, the contributions to pension insurance paid by LTC funds on behalf of informal caregivers help to avoid old-age poverty that might otherwise result from informal caregiving.
- Finally, the introduction of LTCI put the *quality of caregiving* as an issue on to the political agenda. The intense debate led to the LTC Quality Assurance Act (*Pflege-Qualitätssicherungsgesetz*) of 2001. Also, in the recent reform quality is one of the major issues (see below). Since LTCI was introduced, numerous scandals have been publicized, but this should rather be regarded as an indicator for increased attention than as evidence for worsening quality. On the contrary, according to the reports published by the Peak Organization of the Medical Review Boards (MDS), the quality of formal caregiving has improved, though there is still room for more improvement.[14]

Besides those achievements certain *weaknesses* can be identified, which demand improvement in the respective issues:

- The reported decline in family caregiving must be regarded as a sign that *future care arrangements* are an issue of some concern. On the one hand, family caregiving must be stabilized (Döhner and Rothgang 2006); on the other hand, new mixed care arrangements have to be developed and implemented relying on informal care and formal care together with some volunteer work. This implies that families accept 'strangers' as partners in the caregiving process and that professionals find a new role which highlights cooperation with families and counselling as much as hands-on caregiving. It also implies an increasing role for new types of housing (Schmidt 2009).
- Right from the beginning, the *definition of the need for long-term care* was criticized (Wingenfeld 2000; Döhner and Rothgang 2006). The critique particularly focused on people with dementia, whose specific needs are not taken sufficiently into account when the eligibility for benefits is assessed. The assessment is based on the ability to perform activities of daily living but, for example, the permanent need for surveillance which might follow from dementia is not accounted for. In 2001, therefore, a new benefit particularly for people with dementia or similar conditions was introduced, which allows beneficiaries to spend up to an additional €460 per year on services. The amount, however, was so limited that only a minority of those entitled have taken advantage of this benefit,[15] indicating that it missed its target.
- The central weakness of Germany's long-term care insurance has been the *lack of any adjustment* of LTCI benefits. While prices for long-term care services have been increasing LTCI benefits have nominally remained constant for one and a half decades. As a consequence co-payments have

gone up considerably. If a delegitimization of the insurance system is to be prevented, benefits must be adjusted properly.

- Finally, *sustainable financing* must be mentioned. As described in the section on financing, above, the balance sheet has shown deficits for most years of this decade. Even the results shown there, however, have only been possible because of the lack of any adjustment of benefits. Given that for the future adjustment is necessary, either the contribution rate must be increased considerably or additional sources of financing have to be found.

The 2008 Reform

In May 2008 the Long-term Care Further Development Act (*Pflege-Weiterentwicklungsgesetz*) was passed, which took effect on 1 July 2008. The reform mainly tries to improve the delivery side of caregiving or – more precisely – the infrastructural prerequisites for the utilization of services (Igl 2008). Adjustment of benefits and the financing question are also tackled, albeit in a less convincing way. The major contents of this reform Act are:

- the introduction of a new instrument called 'nursing care time' (*Pflegezeit*);
- the promotion of rehabilitation;
- case management and counselling;
- quality improvements;
- adjustment of benefits; and
- financing.

In the following sections each of these areas is addressed in some detail (see also Igl 2008; Rothgang and Preuss 2009, for a more encompassing treatment).

Nursing care time. The basic idea of this instrument is to temporarily release family caregivers from work. According to the Nursing Care Time Act, which was passed as part of the reform, employees may stay absent from work for up to 10 days in order to organize long-term care for a close family member when there is a sudden need for such care. Continuation of payments, however, is only granted if there is respective provision in wage settlements. This has been criticized on the grounds that, for instance, employees receive continued payment if they stay at home to care for a sick child but not if they care for a dependent elderly person. Moreover, employees may stay absent from work for up to six months in order to provide informal care to a close relative ('nursing care time'). The entitlement is only valid against employers with at least 15 employees in order to protect small businesses from disruption. Once again there is neither provision for continuation of payments, nor a respective LTCI benefit as it was originally planned. Nevertheless, LTCI pays contributions to unemployment insurance, health insurance and long-term care insurance for respective caregivers.

Rehabilitation. Although the LTCI Act asks for activating care and although people in need of LTC have a legal entitlement to rehabilitation, rehabilitation is rare for people in need of LTC. In just 6 per cent of all cases the

Medical Review Board recommends rehabilitation (Deutscher Bundestag 2004): gerontologists, on the other hand, claim that the potential for rehabilitation is much higher (Martin *et al.* 2000). This discrepancy is mainly due to disincentives for providers as well as sickness funds, which finance the expenses for rehabilitation (Rothgang 1997: 155 ff.). For formal care providers, successful rehabilitation bears the risk that the care level of the respective client might be downgraded. In nursing homes this means less remuneration, and also in home care the amount of services bought might be reduced as the legal claims of the beneficiary against the LTCI decline in case of downgrading. For funding agencies, an important distinction between health care and long-term care insurance has to be highlighted: though each sickness fund also organizes an LTC fund and though insurees are normally insured against health and LTC risks with the same fund, the two branches operate under distinct frameworks. Sickness funds compete with each other. They receive funding according to the number and risk structure of their insurees. Consequently, the individual sickness fund has to bear the costs for any rehabilitation measure it grants. The savings that may follow from any downgrading in the level of care of an individual client, however, are spread among all long-term care funds as in Social LTCI all expenses are financed from all funds together and these funds do not compete with each other. It is easy to see that funds have no incentive to finance rehabilitation even if it has the potential of reducing long-term care costs significantly.

Thus the 2008 reform has introduced a bonus of €1,536 for nursing homes if – due to rehabilitation – a resident is assessed into a lower level of care. On the other hand, sickness funds have to pay a fine of €2,072 if they do not grant rehabilitation even though it has been recommended by the Medical Review Board. By introducing these monetary incentives government has for the first time acknowledged the prevailing disincentives and tackled the problem. Whether the amount of the bonus/fine is sufficient to change behaviour is still to be seen. The introduction of competition among LTCI funds, on the other hand, would certainly and more directly solve the problem.

Care management and counselling. When suddenly confronted with the need to organize long-term care, families still have difficulties in finding the necessary information to organize a suitable care arrangement (Döhner *et al.* 2008). The improvement of counselling and case management structures has therefore been one of the major targets of the reform. The solution put forward is the founding of so-called *Pflegestützpunkte*, i.e. information centres, where care advisers (*Pflegeberater*) can help to systematically analyse needs, inform about legal claims against LTCI but also other social security systems, and inform about available services in order to finally draw up an individual needs plan (cf. Michel-Auli 2009). Originally the government had planned for a mandatory network of 3,000–4,000 centres, but the federal states vetoed this policy, hinting about already existing counselling structures, which, however, differ greatly among federal states. In the end, the federal government makes about €60 million available to support the introduction of such information centres and the federal states are responsible for the introduction of the structure. Until now, federal states' plans have added up to about 600 information centres, which is much less than originally planed (Rothgang *et al.* 2009; Sendler 2009). By April 2010 only about 250 centres have started to work. On the other hand, all but two federal states joined the programme, which therefore might develop into an important element for strengthening the LTC infrastructure (Schaeffer and Kuhlmey 2008).

Quality improvements. There is no issue that has been given more room in the Reform Act than the issue of quality assurance and quality improvement. Respective new regulations include the obligation of service providers to organize internal quality management, the introduction of expert guidelines, and the introduction of an arbitration board (*Schiedsstelle*) for quality issues. Most important, however, seems to be the quality inspections by the Medical Review Board and the subsequent publication of the results. The Medical Review Boards undertake quality inspections of service providers for both home care and nursing home care. Until recently, however, the frequency was rather low. They performed about 1,000 inspections per year in nursing homes – with about 10,000 existing nursing homes. This frequency will be increased dramatically, and from 2011 onwards each of the nursing homes should see at least one quality inspection a year, which is a tenfold increase on today's frequency. Moreover, until now, the Review Boards were not permitted to publish the results of their inspections. Now they are obliged to publish them in a way comprehensible to the layman. In the meantime LTCI funds and service providers have agreed upon a system of reporting the results of these inspections that uses school grades, which are familiar to everyone. Inspections using the new reporting formulae started in July 2009. Though the system for reporting is highly contested among experts, the potential effect of the resulting competition of service providers seems to be enormous.

Adjustment of benefits. As part of the reform, benefits have been/are to be adjusted thrice – in July 2008, January 2010 and January 2012. The amounts of adjustment are fixed and differentiated according to type of benefit and level of dependency. Table 6 shows the respective amounts for 2007 (before the reform) and for 2012 (after the last step of the adjustment).[16] As the table reveals, adjustment rates are highest for in-kind benefits in home care, while there is no adjustment at all for nursing home care in levels I and II.

Differentiated adjustment rates can be interpreted as an attempt to diminish the gap between benefits in formal home care and formal nursing home care as has been demanded, e.g. in the report by the Commission for Achieving Financial Sustainability for the Social Security Systems (BMGS 2003). On the other hand, adjustment rates are highest for in-kind benefits in home care, which is the area with the lowest spending volume, while there is no adjustment at all for nursing home care in levels I and II – the categories with the highest expenditure in 2007. This already hints at the major problem of this adjustment: its magnitude. On average from 2007 to 2012 benefits are rising nominally by 1.4 per cent per year. This is just sufficient to cover inflation, but there is certainly no compensation for the period until 2008, with massive loss of real purchasing power of LTCI benefits. When related to the period

Table 6

Adjustment of monthly benefits according to type of benefit

	Expenses in 2007 (billion €)	Amount of benefits		Change		Average annual growth rate in % (geometric mean)	
		2007	2012				
	(€)	(€)	(€)	(€)	(%)	2007–2012	1996–2015
Home care: in kind benefits							
Level I	0.8	384	450	66	17.2	3.2	0.8
Level II	1.1	921	1,100	179	19.4	3.6	0.9
Level III	0.5	1,432	1,550	118	8.2	1.6	0.4
Home care: cash benefits							
Level I	1.7	205	235	30	14.6	2.8	0.7
Level II	1.6	410	440	30	7.3	1.4	0.4
Level III	0.7	665	700	35	5.3	1.0	0.3
Nursing home care							
Level I	2.6	1,023	1,023	0	0.0	0.0	0.0
Level II	4.0	1,279	1,279	0	0.0	0.0	0.0
Level III	2.2	1,432 .	1,550	118	8.2	1.6	0.4
Total					*7.1*	*1.4*	*0.4*

Source: Author's calculations, based on Social Code Book XI and data published by the Federal Ministry of Health.
See: www.bmg.bund.de/cln_100/nn_1193090/SharedDocs/Downloads/DE/Statistiken/
Statistiken_20Pflege/xls-Finanzentwicklung-der-sozialen-Pflegeversicherung-Ist-Ergebnisse.html.
www.bmg.bund.de/cln_169/nn_1193090/SharedDocs/Downloads/DE/Pflege/
Informationen/Leistungsempfaenger-Pflegestufen-xls.html.

1996–2015, with the former year marking the start of benefits in nursing home care and the latter the first time when adjustment is reconsidered, the average growth rate is 0.4 per cent per year, which is far below general inflation or inflation for LTC services and therefore marks a considerable loss of real purchasing power.

The reform also commits the government to check every three years whether further adjustment is needed, starting in 2015. Such adjustments must exceed neither general inflation nor wage rises. They are therefore doomed to fall below rises of LTC service prices.[17] Moreover, adjustments are only due if the macro-economic situation permits them. In short: the commitment to further adjustment is fairly weak and far away from an automatic adjustment mechanism, which alone is suitable if purchasing power of LTCI services is to be kept constant and trust in the system is to be reinforced (Rothgang and Igl 2007; Rothgang and Dräther 2009).

Financing. With respect to financing, the Coalition Treaty of 2005 promised the introduction of a demographic reserve fund, i.e. a funded element of financing and at the same time the collection of a contribution from private mandatory LTCI in order to equalize the distinct risk structure of the two insurance systems. In the end, none of these elements was realized, but the contribution rate was raised by 0.25 percentage points. Such an increase in the rate yields additional contributions of about €2.6 billion. On the other hand the reform also produces additional spending: for the adjustment of benefits, for the extension of entitlements for day and night care, for higher benefits for people suffering from dementia, and so on. According to the Reform Bill, these extra expenses add up to €1.04 billion in 2009 and increase up to €2.2 billion in 2012.[18] Financing is therefore said to be secured only until 2014. The Bill explicitly says that beyond that there is no provision for financing further regular adjustments, which are nevertheless necessary. By and large, with respect to financing the reform just buys time – no more and no less.

According to the Bill, financing is secured until 2014. This statement, however, was risky then and should by now be regarded as faulty. The original calculation took into account neither the annual deficit before the reform, which was €320 million in 2007,[19] nor extra expenditures that might result from a new definition of dependency as developed by the Expert Commission initiated by the government (see below). Most important, it could not take into account the economic crisis we are in now. Therefore, with respect to financing the debate about another reform must start earlier than expected, preferably in this legislative period.

The need for reforms after the reform

The above discussion of the 2008 reform has already highlighted some issues that need reconsideration fairly soon. In the following, therefore, perspectives with respect to a new definition of dependency, and financing, are discussed. Apart from that, naturally, the implementation of the recent reform has to be evaluated. For several of the key issues, particularly the information centres, the reports on quality inspections and the incentives for rehabilitation, it is too early to conclude how nearly the targets have been reached.

New definition of dependency. The definition of dependency has been criticized right from the beginning. The benefits for dependent people suffering from dementia, introduced in 2002, did not reach their target. As part of the 2008 reform, therefore, the amount of benefits was increased up to €2,000 a year and the entitlement was extended also to people who are not entitled to other LTCI benefits as the severity of their deficits is not above the threshold. Since the infrastructure for services designed particularly for this target group has also improved, utilization is now increasing. So, from 2007 to 2008 expenditure on these benefits doubled, though the new regulation had only been in place since July 2008.

Nevertheless, this approach seemed to be unsatisfactory as an attempt to correct an inappropriate definition of dependency was made by granting benefits to people not falling under this definition. Therefore, in 2006 an Expert Commission was founded to develop a new concept of dependency and a respected assessment instrument. In January 2009 the Commission reported and presented both a definition, which distinguishes five rather than three levels of dependency, and a respective assessment tool that grasps dependency much better and also explicitly looks into behavioural and cognitive patterns that cause dependency and the need for surveillance (Büscher and Wingenfeld 2009). In May the Commission published a second report dealing with some questions of implementation, but the issue could not be dealt with as the general election stopped all attempts at new legislation. Thus the new definition of dependency and respective entitlements will be a major issue for long-term care policy in the current legislative period.

Financing. Given the greying of German society, the number of people in need of long-term care will increase continuously (cf. Costa-Font *et al.* 2008; Dräther and Holl-Manoharan 2009). Moreover, the changing patterns of utilization and the necessity to adjust benefits will lead to a considerable increase in LTCI expenses as percentage of GDP (Comas-Herrera *et al.* 2006). Within the present system of Social LTCI this yields a doubling of the contribution rate (Rothgang 2002; BMGS 2003; Dräther and Holl-Manoharan 2009). If such an increase is regarded as unacceptable, additional sources for revenue are to be identified. Several proposals have been discussed in the past (cf. Rothgang 2004; Rothgang and Igl 2007). The proposal to fully transform Social LTCI into a private funded system does not stand a real chance as this would result in a much higher fiscal burden for three to four decades. The integration of private and Social LTCI into a 'citizens insurance', which would relieve fiscal pressure from Social LTCI as the risk structure of those in private LTCI is so much better (Rothgang 2010), has also become rather unrealistic since the general election as the parties that form the new government are opposed to it. Therefore, two main options remain: tax financing and the introduction of an additional (funded) component.

Today, in pension insurance about one-third of all revenue is from taxes. This is meant to compensate for those activities of insurance funds that are not closely related to the insured risk and should rather be financed from the general public budget. In 2004, tax financing was also introduced into social health-care insurance and in 2007 it was decided to increase tax financing up to €14 billion, which corresponds to the expenses of children which are insured within the system free of charge. The rationale was that the insurance of children free of charge is a matter of family policy, which should be tax-financed. Similarly, it could be argued that the insurance of children free of charge within Social LTCI also merits a tax subsidy, which could amount up to €0.5 billion. As the grand coalition increased tax financing in health-care insurance it is still possible that the conservatives may also go for a tax grant in LTCI.

Even more likely is the introduction of an element of funding (cf. Rothgang 2009). This could happen either inside or outside the Social LTCI. In the former case the contribution rate simply has to be increased in order to realize a surplus, which can be accumulated. As accumulated public funds are always in danger of being misused once there is an urgent need for revenue in other policy areas, strong legal protection against this would be necessary. Alternatively, a private mandatory supplementary insurance could be introduced, which might be used, for example, to finance adjustment. Respective concepts have been proposed by the private insurance industry and the Christian Social Union of Bavaria (see Rothgang 2009 for details). As the premiums are proposed to be set per capita with no relation to available income and as they are meant to be paid by employees only, this solution would imply certain kinds of redistribution. It also increases administrative costs as another player would have to be integrated into collective bargaining processes. It is therefore not clear that such a proposal will get through.

By and large, it is therefore too early to know what might happen in this parliamentary session. However, there is certainly the need for some kind of financing reform.

Conclusion

So, reconsidering the above analysis: What can be learned? First, the introduction of long-term care insurance in Germany led to the complete coverage of the whole population in an insurance system. Introduced as a pay-as-you-go system, LTCI was able to grant benefits immediately. Public spending has been increased and the capacities for formal caregiving have been growing ever since then. Quality issues have become prominent and family care was supported along with formal care. For a decade and a half the system worked with a constant contribution rate – although due to demographic change the number of beneficiaries has increased enormously.

The latter, however, was only possible as capped benefits have not been adjusted and therefore the real purchasing power has declined considerably. In other words, the German example demonstrates that the contribution rate in any pay-as-you-go insurance system will increase if the number of elderly is increasing – as is the case in all Western European countries – and benefits are adjusted properly. The German example particularly highlights difficulties that arise once contributions are not levied on the whole income but just on income from gainful employment (and derived social benefits as unemployment benefits and pensions) and this part of the income grows more slowly than the GDP.

In particular, the German case demonstrates that:

- it is important to insure the whole population in one integrated system, as the existence of more than one system (such as Social LTCI and mandatory private LTCI) raises unresolved questions of fairness, particularly if the risk structure between both branches of the insurance differs as much as it does in Germany;
- contributions should be levied on all income so as to avoid fiscal turbulence once the structure of the functional income distribution changes;
- in a pay-as-you-go system a growing contribution rate is to be expected as the number of elderly persons increases;
- it is possible to create legitimacy for capped benefits if there is provision for proper adjustment, which should relate to macro-economic variables such as inflation and wages;

- interfaces with health-care services and other services have to be organized, which includes a competitive organization of LTCI once health-care insurance is competitive;
- individual choice increases acceptance of the system but must go together with counselling and case management structures;
- it is important to have a definition of entitlement that does not exclude either physically or mentally ill persons.

In this sense the German experience demonstrates the strengths and weaknesses of a Social LTCI and gives some clues about what should be avoided and how certain problems might be solved.

Notes

1. The Netherlands can be regarded as a forerunner, as a long-term care insurance (AWBZ) had already been introduced in 1968 (see Schut and Van den Berg, this volume).
2. See e.g. Economic Policy Committee and DG ECFIN (2006) and OECD (2007) for some recent projections.
3. Those figures are based on the current German definition of the need for long-term care, which is comparatively strict (see Rothgang and Comas-Herrera 2003).
4. See Pabst and Rothgang (2000) for the situation before LTCI was introduced.
5. By the end of 2006, some 213,000 residents of nursing homes received social assistance (BMG 2008). At that time about 628,000 people resided in nursing homes, with 578,000 of them being in need of long-term care.
6. These figures are based on the author's calculations based on data from the Department of Health for 2008 (www.bmg.bund.de/cln_160/nn_1193090/SharedDocs/Downloads/DE/Statistiken/Statistiken_20Pflege/Leistungsempfaenger-Jahresende-Altersgruppen,templateId=raw,property=publicationFile.pdf/Leistungsempfaenger-Jahresende-Altersgruppen.pdf).
7. The amount of contributions differs according to the level of dependency of the person cared for and the time spent caring. Contributions to pension funds require a minimum of 14 hours of care a week. The minimum contribution paid is equivalent to 26.7 per cent of the contribution paid for a full-time employee with average salary, while the maximum is 80 per cent of this amount.
8. The employers' part is tax-free. In order to compensate employers, 15 out of 16 provinces abolished one bank holiday. In Saxony, no bank holiday was abolished and thus employees bear the first percentage point of the contribution on their own and only the additional contribution is equally shared between employers and employees.
9. Figures for 2007 and 2008 are misleading as adjustments in the statistical procedures lead to a slight overestimation of respective numbers.
10. According to a representative survey conducted in 2002, apart from about 2 million recipients of LTCI benefits, there are about 3 million older people who need help, mainly with iADLs, but do not qualify for LTCI benefits (Schneekloth and Leven 2003: 7).
11. Federal Ministry of Health. Figures available at: www.bmg.bund.de/cln_160/nn_1193090/SharedDocs/Downloads/DE/Pflege/Informationen/Leistungsempfaenger-Pflegestufen-xls.html.
12. In 1995, a loan of €560 million was given to the central government, which paid it back without interest in 2002.

13. The private mandatory insurance is funded: in order to accumulate funds for old age, premiums in younger age are higher than necessary to cover the current risk. Since private LTCI was legally obliged also to grant benefits for people already in need of long-term care and to sell insurance to the older old with capped premiums, there is also an element of pay-as-you-go within this system as younger cohorts subsidize older cohorts (see Wasem 2000 for details). The ability of private insurance companies to build up a capital stock, though, is due to the much better risk structure of their insurees, which produce only half as much costs as members of social insurance (Dräther *et al.* 2009).

14. The MDS published its first report on the quality of formal caregiving in 2004 and the second in 2007. In the latter, progress was reported, but on a level that is still partly unsatisfactory.

15. In the Bill the number of potential beneficiaries was estimated at 500,000 (500,000 to 550,000). If all of them were to claim benefits of €460, annual expenses would be €230–253 million. In reality, until 2007 annual expenses for this benefit have been around €20–30 million. This means that only one in ten potential beneficiaries made use of it.

16. Amounts of benefits have also been adjusted for fiscally minor benefits such as day and night care, whose benefits are linked to the major home care benefits. While until 2008 utilization of day and night care diminished entitlement to in-kind and in-cash benefits, now claims for day and night care are partly on top. Extra benefits for people suffering from dementia have also been extended (see below, section on the need for reforms after the reform).

17. The Commission for Achieving Financial Sustainability for the Social Security Systems has instead argued for an adjustment formula as a weighted mean of inflation and nominal wage development (BMGS 2003).

18. For 2009, Social LTCI shows a surplus of about €1 billion. Given the above-mentioned extra expenditure, for 2012 the system would once again show a deficit.

19. For 2008, extra contributions of €1.3 billion were projected. If the extra expenditures are subtracted a surplus of €0.82 billion follows. In reality the surplus was €0.63 billion, leaving a gap between projection and reality of €200 million – even before the economic crisis hit the system.

References

Augurzky, B., Borchert, L., Deppisch, R., Krolop, S., Mennicken, R., Preuss, M., Rothgang, H., Stocker-Müller, M. and Wasem, J. (2008), *Heimentgelte bei der stationären Pflege in Nordrhein-Westfalen. Ein Bundesländervergleich* [Nursing home reimbursement in North Rhine-Westphalia], RWI-Materialien, Heft 44, Essen: Rheinisch-Westfälisches Institut für Wirtschaftsforschung.

BMG (Bundesministerium für Gesundheit) (2008), *4. Bericht über die Entwicklung der Pflegebedürftigkeit* [4th report on the development of long-term care], Berlin: BMG.

BMGS (Bundesministerium für Gesundheit und Soziale Sicherung) (ed.) (2003), *Nachhaltigkeit in der Finanzierung der sozialen Sicherungssysteme. Bericht der Kommission* [Sustainability of social security financing: commission report], Berlin: Eigenverlag.

Büscher, A. and Wingenfeld, K. (2009), Pflegebedürftigkeit und Pflegeleistungen. In H. Dräther, K. Jacobs and H. Rothgang (eds), *Fokus Pflegeversicherung. Nach der Reform ist vor der Reform* [Focus LTC insurance: after the reform is before the reform], Berlin: KomPart-Verlag, pp. 257–81.

Comas-Herrera, A., Wittenberg, R., Costa-Font, J., Gori, C., diMaio, A., Patxot, C., Pickard, L., Pozzi, A. and Rothgang, H. (2006), Future long-term care expenditure in Germany, Spain, Italy and the United Kingdom, *Ageing and Society*, 26: 285–302.

Costa-Font, J., Wittenberg, R., Patxot, C., Comas-Herrera, A., Gori, C., di Maio, A., Pickard, L., Pozzi, A. and Rothgang, H. (2008), Projecting long-term care expenditure in four European Union member states: the influence of demographic scenarios, *Social Indicators Research*, 86: 303–21.

Deutscher Bundestag (2004), Dritter Bericht über die Entwicklung der Pflegeversicherung [3rd report on the development of long-term care]. Available at: www.bmg.bund.de/cln_040/nn_773126/SharedDocs/Publikationen/Pflege/a-503, templateId=raw,property=publicationFile.pdf/a-503.pdf (accessed 19 May 2008).

Döhner, H. and Rothgang, H. (2006), Pflegebedürftigkeit. Zur Bedeutung der familialen Pflege für die Sicherung der Langzeitpflege [Need of long-term care: the role of informal family caregiving for securing long-term care], *Bundesgesundheitsblatt – Gesundheitsforschung – Gesundheitsschutz*, 49, 6: 583–94.

Döhner, H., Kofahl, C., Lüdecke, D. and Mnich, E. (eds) (2008), *Family Care for Older People in Germany*, Results from the European Project EUROFAMCARE, Münster: LIT.

Dräther, H. and Holl-Manoharan, N. (2009), Modellrechnungen zum zukünftigen Finanzierungsbedarf der sozialen Pflegeversicherung. In H. Dräther, K. Jacobs and H. Rothgang (eds), *Fokus Pflegeversicherung. Nach der Reform ist vor der Reform* [Focus LTC insurance: after the reform is before the reform], Berlin: KomPart-Verlag, pp. 13–40.

Dräther, H., Jacobs, K. and Rothgang, H. (2009), Pflege-Bürgerversicherung. In H. Dräther, K. Jacobs and H. Rothgang (eds), *Fokus Pflegeversicherung. Nach der Reform ist vor der Reform* [Focus LTC insurance: after the reform is before the reform], Berlin: KomPart-Verlag, pp. 71–93.

Economic Policy Committee and DG ECFIN (2006), *The Impact of Ageing on Public Expenditure: Projections for the EU25 Member States on Pensions, Health Care, Long-term Care, Education and Unemployment Transfers (2004–2050)*, Special Report 1/2006, Brussels.

Igl, G. (2008), Das Gesetz zur strukturellen Weiterentwicklung der Pflegeversicherung [The Long-term Care Further Development Act], *Neue Juristische Wochenschrift*, 31: 2214–19.

Jacobs, K. (1995), Zur Kohärenz von gesetzlicher Pflegeversicherung und anderen Zweigen der Sozialversicherung. In U. Fachinger and H. Rothgang (eds), *Die Wirkungen des Pflege-Versicherungsgesetzes* [The impacts of the LTC insurance Act], Berlin: Duncker and Humblot, pp. 245–262.

Martin, S., Zimprich, D., Oster, P., Wahl, H.-W., Minnemann, E., Baethe, M., Grün, U. and Martin, P. (2000), Erfolg und Erfolgsvariabilität stationärer Rehabilitation alter Menschen: Eine empirische Studie auf der Basis medizinisch-geriatrischer und psychosozialer Indikatoren [Success and the variability of success of hospital-based rehabilitation of old people: an empirical study on the basis of medico-geriatric and psychosocial indicators], *Zeitschrift für Gerontologie und Geriatrie*, 33: 24–35.

Michel-Auli, P. (2009), Pflegeberatung und Pflegestützpunkte – Eine neue Form der wohnortbezogenen Beratung und Versorgung. In H. Dräther, K. Jacobs and H. Rothgang (eds), *Fokus Pflegeversicherung. Nach der Reform ist vor der Reform* [Focus LTC insurance: after the reform is before the reform], Berlin: KomPart-Verlag, pp. 155–73.

OECD (2007), *Trends in Severe Disability Among Elderly People*, DELSA/HEA/WD/ HWP.

Österle, A. and Rothgang, H. (2010), Long-term care. In H. Obinger, C. Pierson, F. Castles and S. Leibfried (eds), *The Oxford Handbook of Comparative Welfare States*, Oxford: Oxford University Press, pp. 405–18.

Pabst, S. and Rothgang, H. (2000), Die Einführung der Pflegeversicherung. In S. Leibfried and U. Wagschal (eds), *Bilanzen, Reformen und Perspektiven des deutschen*

Sozialstaats [Results, reforms and perspectives of the German welfare state], Frankfurt: Campus, pp. 340–77.

Pavolini, E. and Ranci, C. (2008), Restructuring the welfare state: reforms in long-term care in Western European countries, *Journal of European Social Policy*, 18: 246–59.

Roth, G. and Rothgang, H. (2001), Sozialhilfe und Pflegebedürftigkeit: Analyse der Zielerreichung und Zielverfehlung der Gesetzlichen Pflegeversicherung nach fünf Jahren [Social welfare and the need for long-term care: analysis of achievements and failures of the statutory LTC insurance after five years], *Zeitschrift für Gerontologie und Geriatrie*, 34, 4: 292–305.

Rothgang, H. (1997), Ziele und Wirkungen der Pflegeversicherung. Eine ökonomische Analyse [Aims and effects of Germany's long-term care insurance: an economic analysis], *Schriften des Zentrums für Sozialpolitik*, 7, Frankfurt: Campus.

Rothgang, H. (2002), Finanzwirtschaftliche und strukturelle Entwicklungen in der Pflegeversicherung bis 2040 und mögliche alternative Konzepte. In Enquete Kommission 'Demographischer Wandel' des Deutschen Bundestags (ed.), *Herausforderungen unser älter werdenden Gesellschaft an den einzelnen und die Politik* [Challenges of our ageing society for individuals and politics], Studienprogramm, Heidelberg: R. V. Decker, pp. 1–254.

Rothgang, H. (2004), Reformoptionen zur Finanzierung der Pflegesicherung – Darstellung und Bewertung [Reform options for the financing of long-term care insurance: description and assessment], *Zeitschrift für Sozialreform*, 50, 6: 584–616.

Rothgang, H. (2009), Einführung von Kapitaldeckung in der sozialen Pflegeversicherung. In H. Dräther, K. Jacobs and H. Rothgang (eds), *Fokus Pflegeversicherung. Nach der Reform ist vor der Reform* [Focus LTC insurance: after the reform is before the reform], Berlin: KomPart-Verlag, pp. 95–121.

Rothgang, H. (2010), Gerechtigkeit im Verhältnis von Sozialer Pflegeversicherung und Privater Pflegepflichtversicherung [Fairness in Germany's long-term care insurance: the relationship between social insurance and private mandatory insurance], *Das Gesundheitswesen*, 72, 3: 154–60.

Rothgang, H. and Comas-Herrera, A. (2003), Dependency rates and health expectancy. In A. Comas-Herrera and R. Wittenberg (eds), *European Study of Long-Term Care Expenditure: Report to the Employment and Social Affairs DG of the European Commission*, PSSRU Discussion Paper 1840, London: London School of Economics, pp. 159–78.

Rothgang, H. and Dräther, H. (2009), Zur aktuellen Diskussion über die Finanzsituation der Sozialen Pflegeversicherung. In H. Dräther, K. Jacobs and H. Rothgang (eds), *Fokus Pflegeversicherung. Nach der Reform ist vor der Reform* [Focus LTC insurance: after the reform is before the reform], Berlin: KomPart-Verlag, pp. 41–69.

Rothgang, H. and Igl, G. (2007), Long-term care in Germany, *Japanese Journal of Social Security Policy*, 6, 1: 54–84.

Rothgang, H. and Preuss, M. (2009), Bisherige Erfahrungen und Defizite der Pflegeversicherung und die Reform 2008 aus sozialpolitischer Sicht. In K.-J. Bieback (ed.), *Die Reform der Pflegeversicherung 2008* [The 2008 reform of LTC insurance], Münster: Lit-Verlag, pp. 7–39.

Rothgang, H., Borchert, L., Müller, R. and Unger, R. (2008), *GEK-Pflegereport 2008. Medizinische Versorgung in Pflegeheimen* [GEK report on long-term care 2008: medical care in nursing homes], GEK-Edition Band 66, St Augustin: Asgard-Verlag.

Rothgang, H., Kulik, D., Müller, R. and Unger, R. (2009), *GEK-Pflegereport 2009. Regionale Unterschiede in der Versorgung* [GEK report on long-term care 2009: regional differences in long-term care], GEK-Edition Band 66, St Augustin: Asgard-Verlag.

Schaeffer, D. and Kuhlmey, A. (2008), Pflegestützpunkte – Impuls zur Weiterentwicklung der Pflege [Care information: stimulus for development of long-term care], *Zeitschrift für Gerontologie und Geriatrie*, 41: S. 81–5.

Schmidt, R. (2009), Veränderungen von Pflegearrangements: Neue Pflege- und spezielle Wohnformen. In H. Dräther, K. Jacobs and H. Rothgang (eds), *Fokus Pflegeversicherung. Nach der Reform ist vor der Reform* [Focus LTC insurance: after the reform is before the reform], Berlin: KomPart-Verlag, pp. 301–29.

Schneekloth, U. and Leven, I. (2003): Hilfe- und Pflegebedürftige in Privathaushalten in Deutschland 2002. Schnellbericht. Erste Ergebnisse der Repräsentativerhebung im Rahmen des Forschungsprojekts 'Möglichkeiten und Grenzen einer selbständigen Lebensführung hilfe- und pflegebedürftiger Menschen in privaten Haushalten' (MuG 3) Im Auftrag des Bundesministeriums für Familie, Senioren, Frauen und Jugend. Bonn: BMFSFJ. Available at: www.bmfsfj.de/RedaktionBMFSFJ/Abteilung3/Pdf-Anlagen/hilfe-und-pflegebeduerftige-in-privathaushalten.

Sendler, J. (2009), Wie steht es um die Einrichtung von Pflegestützpunkten? [How about care information centres?], *Soziale Sicherheit*, 7–8: 270–4.

StBA (Statistisches Bundesamt) (2009a), *Pflegestatistik 2007. Pflege im Rahmen der Pflegeversicherung* [Statistics of long-term care 2007], 4. Bericht. Ländervergleiche – Pflegeheime, Wiesbaden: Statistisches Bundesamt.

StBA (Statistisches Bundesamt) (2009b), *Pflegestatistik 2007. Pflege im Rahmen der Pflegeversicherung. Deutschlandergebnisse* [Statistics of long-term care 2007], Wiesbaden: Statistisches Bundesamt.

Wasem, J. (2000), Die private Pflegepflichtversicherung – ein Modell für eine alternative Organisation der sozialen Sicherung zwischen Markt und Staat? In W. Schmähl (ed.), *Soziale Sicherung zwischen Markt und Staat* [Social security between market and the state], Schriften des Vereins für Socialpolitik, Neue Folge, Band 275, Berlin: Duncker and Humblot, pp. 79–110.

Wingenfeld, K. (2000), Pflegebedürftigkeit, Pflegebedarf und pflegerische Leistungen. In B. Rennen-Althoff and D. Schaeffer (eds), *Handbuch Pflegewissenschaft* [Handbook of nursing sciences], Weinheim: Juventa, pp. 339–61.

6

Long-term Care in Central and South-Eastern Europe: Challenges and Perspectives in Addressing a 'New' Social Risk

August Österle

Introduction

In recent years, social policy analysis has started to focus more on developments in Central and South-Eastern Europe (CSEE), both in single country studies and in comparative studies attempting to connect regional experiences with comparative social policy analysis and with the literature on welfare state models (e.g. Cerami 2006; Fenger 2007; Castles and Obinger 2008; Hacker 2009). In all of these efforts, long-term care (LTC) has been largely neglected. This neglect is also a reflection of the role that LTC plays in the national welfare policies and policy debates. In the CSEE region, as in Mediterranean countries, help and support in the case of LTC needs largely remain a family responsibility. Existing social policy approaches are characterized by social assistance orientation, fragmentation and low levels of infrastructure development. Broader and more focused debates on the future of care systems in this region are also being hindered by a lack of data and information and large variations in the way populations generally understand and conceptualize care. There is very little focused research on long-term care within countries, and the region is almost non-existent in the international comparative LTC literature.

Over the past two decades, many European countries have started to substantially extend existing social protection schemes, or to implement new ones, against the risk of dependency (e.g. Ungerson and Yeandle 2007; Doyle and Timonen 2008; Österle and Rothgang 2010). In this process, many countries have introduced novel approaches. Examples include the national system of long-term care that came into effect in Spain in 2007 (see Costa-Font, this volume), long-term care insurance introduced in Germany in 1995 (see Rothgang, this volume) or a cash for care-centred approach introduced in Austria in 1993 (Österle 2010). This chapter asks whether countries in CSEE follow this broader European trend of major, partly path-departing long-term care reforms. Given the social policy transformations taking place in other welfare sectors in this region in the past twenty years and recognizing the importance of principles such as decentralization, privatization or pluralization in this process, reform developments might be expected in the LTC field.

In exploring the question, the chapter provides a review of the reform context and the current situation of LTC in the CSEE region, studying developments in the light of the major principles underlying the transition process and discussing key features of current developments in terms of their potential for establishing a new paradigm in LTC policies. The findings of the chapter show that countries in this region share many of the related challenges with other European regions, but they are also confronted with particular parameters that have hindered the realization of more comprehensive LTC systems. Putting the features into a regional and a European comparative perspective and establishing a link with theoretical and conceptual approaches will contribute to a better understanding of LTC developments in this part of Europe. And it will help that the question of long-term care will be included within the growing corpus of literature on social policy in this European region.

The study is based on an international comparative project covering seven CSEE countries: Croatia, the Czech Republic, Hungary, Romania, Serbia, Slovakia and Slovenia. In the following section, the chapter begins with a discussion of the particular demographic and socio-economic developments in the region, and their implications for the future need for long-term care and for alternative modes of providing and financing it. Then, following a brief survey of social policies and social policy transformation in CSEE, the chapter outlines the status quo of the social policies and welfare state provisions for long-term care. In the sections which then follow, the author will delve into an in-depth discussion of three major issues. First, the fragmentation of welfare policies is closely related to issues of (de)centralization, and specifically the often blurred dividing lines between the health and social care sectors. Second, despite the emphasis on pluralization and privatization in the transition process, private sector initiatives are growing slowly in the long-term care sector. Third, the author's discussion will focus on the central role of the family in care systems. In the concluding section, the author discusses the LTC reform process and the perspectives for future LTC policies in the region.

Ageing Societies and Long-term Care Needs in CSEE

Ageing has become one of the major socio-economic concerns in Europe and beyond and an important driver of the debate on the future of long-term care and the financing of that care (e.g. Timonen 2009). According to Eurostat forecasts, in the EU27, the proportion of the population aged 65+ will increase from its current level of 16.9 per cent (2007) to 20.7 per cent in 2020 and 28.2 per cent in 2040. The proportion of those aged 80+ will increase from 4.3 per cent (2007) to 5.8 per cent in 2020 and 9.2 per cent in 2040. These increases are a Europe-wide trend, even though elderly age groups are relatively smaller in Central and Eastern European countries. In the EU10 group, the 2004

Table 1

Demography and long-term care dependency in Central and South-Eastern Europe

		CR	CZ	HU	RO	SE	SK	SLO	EU27
% of	2007	17.0	14.4	15.9	14.9	17.5	11.9	15.9	16.9
population > 65									
Projected % of	2020	19.9	20.8	20.4	17.1	20.3	16.3	20.4	20.7
population > 65	2040	24.9	26.7	28.2	24.9	23.0	24.1	28.4	28.2
% of	2007	3.1	3.3	3.6	2.7	2.7	2.5	3.4	4.3
population > 80									
Projected % of	2020	4.6	4.0	4.7	4.0	5.0	3.1	5.1	5.8
population > 80	2040	7.0	8.1	8.5	6.8	6.7	7.1	9.1	9.2
Life expectancy	total	76	77	73	73	73	74	78	
at birth in years	female	79	80	78	76	76	78	82	
(2006)	male	72	73	69	69	71	70	74	
% of population	2000	5.1	5.1	5.2	5.0	4.9	4.8	5.2	
requiring daily	2020	5.5	5.8	5.7	5.4	5.4	5.4	5.9	
care[a]	2040	5.7	6.4	6.1	5.9	5.8	6.1	6.5	
Long-term care	2000	8.3	7.9	8.2	8.0	8.0	7.4	8.0	
dependency ratio[b]	2020	9.4	9.8	9.4	8.6	8.9	8.7	10.0	
	2040	10.5	12.7	11.7	10.8	10.3	11.0	13.2	

[a]Proportion of total population requiring daily care.
[b]Ratio between total number of dependent people and total number of persons aged 15–59.
Source: Eurostat database (2009a); WHO (2009). See also the Statistical Office of Croatia 2007 (population projection data for 2021 and 2041); and Serbian Academy of Sciences 2007.

accession countries, the proportion of those aged 80 years and older will rise from 2.8 per cent in 2007 to 8.4 per cent in 2040. In three of the new EU member countries, Slovenia, Slovakia and Poland, the proportion of those aged 80+ will more than triple over that period. Somewhat different developments are expected for the South-Eastern European region. Both in Croatia and in Serbia, the proportion of those aged 65+ was even beyond the European average in 2007. In 2040, this age group will account for 24.9 per cent of the population in Croatia, and 23.0 per cent in Serbia, compared to an EU25 average of 28.2 per cent (see table 1).

There are several factors underlying these demographic changes, including developments in life expectancy, in fertility rates, and in migration patterns. For many years, fertility rates in Europe, defined as the number of children per woman in her total lifetime, have been well below the replacement rate of approximately 2.1 children. In 2006, fertility rates ranged between 1.24 in Slovakia and 2.0 in France. While there have been small increases in some Western European countries in recent years, fertility rates are now declining further in Eastern European countries, giving rise to an average fertility rate which is below the Western European average (Eurostat 2009a). In terms of mortality and morbidity, the situation improved in Central Europe beginning in the early 1990s and in Romania and Bulgaria beginning in the later 1990s.

Though gaps in life expectancy are narrowing, they are still about four to five years (McKee *et al.* 2004; Zatonski 2007; Mete 2008). In 2006, average life expectancy in Central-Eastern and South-Eastern Europe ranged from 76 to 80 years for women and from 69 to 73 years for men, compared to 81 to 85 years for women and 74 to 79 years for men in the Western European countries, with Slovenia belonging to this latter group in terms of life expectancy (see table 1).

Even if there are still significant differences seen in life expectancy across Europe, the implications for health and long-term care are quite similar across the continent, as those implications are determined not so much by absolute age, but by periods of ill health, chronic illness or disability. According to WHO estimates, about 5 per cent of the total population are currently in need of daily care. In the study region, this proportion varies between 4.8 per cent in Slovakia and 5.2 per cent in Slovenia. In 2040, the proportion of those needing care in these countries will be between 5.7 and 6.5 per cent (see table 1). Given current and forecast age and morbidity structures, it is undisputed that long-term care needs will increase over the coming four decades. However, the question of the extent of that increase is controversial. According to the Economic Policy Committee and European Commission (2006), the number of people in need of long-term care in a pure ageing scenario, assuming an expansion of morbidity, will double by 2050, whereas (assuming the more optimistic scenario of a compression of morbidity) it will increase by just 31 per cent over the same period. Recent surveys on self-perceived health also confirm the relatively large burden of chronic illness and long-term care needs within the Central-Eastern and South-Eastern European region. Even though cultural differences are important in response behaviour, survey respondents in Eastern and South-Eastern European countries report bad or very bad health status significantly more often. Such health status reports largely correlate with chronic illness or conditions limiting respondents' daily activities (Eurostat 2009b).

Apart from demographic changes affecting long-term care needs, the increase of the elderly population relative to the employment-age population will challenge traditional modes of funding social protection schemes and of caregiving within family networks. The long-term care dependency ratio – the relation between the total number of those in need of care and the population aged 15 to 59 – points towards these implications (see table 1). In 2000, the long-term care dependency ratio ranged between 6.4 per cent in Ireland and 9.9 per cent in Malta and between 7.3 per cent and 8.3 per cent in the study region. According to WHO forecasts, in 2040 the ratio will peak at 14.1 per cent in Malta and 13.2 per cent in Slovenia. In Croatia and in Serbia, in line with the above cited demographic forecasts, the ratio will be just about 10 per cent in 2040.

Ageing societies are not the only challenge to traditional ways of organizing and providing care – there are challenges due to a range of broader socio-demographic and socio-economic developments. The role of the family is central in covering long-term care needs in the CSEE region, both in the way individuals perceive their responsibilities (see table 2) and in the need for individuals to provide that care themselves due to a lack of alternative care

Table 2

Long-term care in Central and South-Eastern Europe: preferences and perceptions

		CR	CZ	HU	RO	SK	SLO	EU27
Care	Home – relative	48	54	66	48	50	43	45
preferences	Home – care service	13	11	8	16	18	15	24
	Home – personal carer	10	9	6	10	13	10	12
	Home of family	10	6	6	10	7	9	5
	Institution	15	16	10	6	7	20	8
	No answer	4	4	4	10	5	3	6
Perceived	Easy	18	18	22	19	22	23	39
access to nursing homes[a]	Difficult	59	65	55	33	57	49	28
Perceived	Easy	25	33	31	24	32	33	41
access to care services[a]	Difficult	50	47	45	39	50	35	25
Perceived responsibilities	Obligatory insurance	76	77	54	74	80	72	70
to pay[b]	Children should pay	88	59	46	67	57	60	48
	House should be sold	58	24	26	27	22	52	25

[a]Perceived access to nursing homes and care services (response categories: very easy, fairly easy (easy); very difficult, fairly difficult (difficult)); agreement in %.
[b]Perceived responsibilities for provision and financing of long-term care (response categories: totally agree, tend to agree (agree); totally disagree, tend to disagree (disagree)); agreement in %.
Source: European Commission (2007).

options (Österle 2010). According to the Eurobarometer survey 2002, about 23 per cent of Europeans provide informal care. In the new EU member states, informal long-term care provision is at slightly higher levels than in the EU average. These differences become more pronounced for caregiving provided within households. By contrast with an EU average of 11 per cent of people providing informal care within the household, the proportion in Hungary, Romania, the Czech Republic, Poland or Bulgaria exceeds 14 per cent (Alber and Köhler 2004).

A trend away from intergenerational cohabitation, increases in single elderly households, increases in employment levels in particular among women and increases in employment-related migration, increases in retirement age and stricter links between regular employment and social security are putting pressure on traditional informal care arrangements. All of these trends are relevant, if indeed not more significant, within the CSEE region. Increasing employment levels and a higher average age of exiting from the labour force, both indicators that are currently below EU average, will reduce the potential for informal caregiving. Significant migration flows from rural into urban areas as well as migration flows towards Western European countries have already increased pressure on governments to find alternatives to traditional family-oriented care arrangements. In future, it is unlikely that families and other informal networks will be in a position to provide similar amounts of informal care (Österle 2010). Taken together, increasing long-term care needs and the changing context for traditional informal care will intensify the pressure on governments to develop new forms of funding and providing long-term care in coming years. The developments and perspectives for long-term care in the region will be discussed in the following sections.

Welfare State Approaches to Dealing with the Risk of Long-term Care

Across Europe, the welfare state has been late in addressing the issue of long-term care. While welfare systems have developed comprehensive schemes for coverage in case of illness, unemployment or loss of income in old age, long-term care has been largely organized, provided and funded within family or other informal networks, and in many countries this still is the case today. Apart from the Nordic European countries, which have taken earlier and more universal approaches towards the risk of dependency, it is only in the past two decades that many European countries have started to substantially extend already existing social protection schemes towards the risk of dependency, or to implement new ones (e.g. Ungerson and Yeandle 2007; Doyle and Timonen 2008; Österle and Rothgang 2010). These new developments have expanded public responsibilities for social protection coverage, while at the same time clarifying individual and/or family responsibilities, in particular in financial terms. In other European countries, not least in Central-Eastern and South-Eastern Europe, public support for long-term care remains very limited and is characterized by fragmentation and an orientation towards providing social assistance. Across the region, there are declarations and policy proposals (e.g. European Commission 2009a; Österle 2010), but these have not yet led to the implementation of long-term care systems that would ensure extended personal and material coverage.

The status quo is also reflected in comparative data on LTC expenditure. Accurate quantitative cross-country comparisons in LTC are still hindered by variations in how each country defines its LTC expenditures, by national differences in the range of services that are covered by those definitions, by national differences in classifying health and social care expenditures or simply because of the lack of systematically collected data. Despite large variations and gaps in published data on public expenditures for long-term care, existing datasets at least provide some general indications of the relative levels of expenditures. Pursuant to data published by OECD and Eurostat, there are only a few countries where LTC expenditures exceed 1.5 per cent of GDP, most notably Denmark and Sweden. In a second group of European countries, expenditures account for between 1 and 1.5 per cent of GDP, including Austria, France, Germany and the United Kingdom. In the CSEE countries, LTC expenditures account for less than 0.5 per cent of GDP.

In the past two decades, the welfare systems in CSEE countries have undergone major transitions, marked by the fall of the communist regimes in Central-Eastern Europe, the disintegration of the former Yugoslavia and the war period in that region. Social policy developments during the transition period have been characterized by reform activities driven by a multiplicity of factors: the search for a new social contract, the disintegration of the previous systems and earlier social safety nets, opposing political ideologies and recommendations of international organizations, but also pressures arising from economic situations that deteriorated for large parts of the populations in the early years of the transformation (Inglot 2008). The region has been identified as a distinctive post-communist welfare state model (Castles and Obinger 2008) or as a hybrid system with pre-communist, communist and post-communist features (Cerami 2006). While the centre of the new welfare systems is characterized by a social insurance orientation, countries are following very different paths within that context (e.g. Cerami 2006; Hacker 2009). In the Czech Republic, for example, social insurance involves strong universal elements and has, in the recent past, incorporated neo-liberal elements, but more by decay than by an explicit policy choice in that direction (Saxonberg and Sirovatka 2009). In South-Eastern Europe, for example in Croatia, welfare reform processes are embedded in the process of state-building, the construction of national identity, the search for defining roles of state actors on central and decentralized levels, and, more recently, pressures to privatize care (Stubbs and Zrinščak 2009). During the entire period from 1990 to the present, long-term care did not play any prominent role in social policy reforms and was widely ignored as a social risk. Debates on long-term care have emerged in small expert groups, and experts from the governmental and non-governmental sectors have put forward policy proposals and even detailed reform documents. But, with a few exceptions, those proposals have not led to broader public debates (Österle 2010). It is only in the very recent past that ageing and long-term care dependency are being more specifically recognized in public policy debates, not least in the context of national strategies addressing the challenges arising from ageing societies, and in connection with the Open Method of Coordination in the European Union (European Commission 2009a).

Considered from a historical perspective, the provision of residential care in CSEE, as in other European countries, has been the major and often sole public response to long-term care needs, even though this has been at generally lower levels relative to Northern and Western European countries. To date, given the lack of alternative care arrangements outside families, residential care has often remained the only alternative if family and other informal care networks are not available. In Croatia, Romania, Serbia and Slovakia, the residential bed density is below 30 beds per 1,000 population aged 65+, in the Czech Republic, Hungary and Slovenia it is between 30 and 60 beds per 1,000 population aged 65+ (Österle 2010). However, these figures do not fully reflect availability. Apart from general data quality concerns, long-term care beds might also be provided in the health sector, and might either be officially declared to be chronic care beds or declared to be acute care beds that are actually used as chronic care beds. Figures from different sources, therefore, point to significant variations in bed density, but they do nothing to change the general picture of medium to low levels of availability in the CSEE region. A low level of bed density, however, is not necessarily correlated with longer waiting lists. Countries with relatively large numbers of residential care beds, such as Slovenia and the Czech Republic, both report long waiting lists (Österle 2010). This points both to stronger growth at present in these countries, in terms of the demand for care from outside households, and it also highlights a lack of community care services that could at least partly cover that need. The Eurobarometer survey 2007 confirms this information, as a relatively small proportion of the population in Slovenia and the Czech Republic considers it easy to obtain access to residential care settings, while in both countries the populace expresses a higher preference for being cared for in long-term care institutions than the EU27 average (see table 2, and European Commission 2007).

Compared to institutional care settings, availability of social services provided in the community is even more limited and fragmented. As a consequence, there is an extreme scarcity of information collected systematically at the country level, and it does not permit quantitative comparisons across countries. From a general perspective, the availability of services provided by the health sector is more widespread. However, those services cover only medically oriented nursing care and are usually provided for a limited period of time only. In the social care sector, community care services developed slowly during the communist regime in the Czech Republic or Hungary (Munday and Lane 1998), whereas in Romania, they did not exist at that time (Dobre 2009). In the transformation process, the governments introduced new regulatory frameworks and a decentralization of responsibilities. However, because of a lack of resources and a lack of political will to systematically develop the social service sector, the availability of care in the community remains at very low levels (Dobre 2009; Ripka and Mareš 2009). Services are usually more widespread in the capital cities and other urban areas. In some rural areas, local initiatives or pilot projects have been developed; in many remote areas, however, community services are non-existent (Österle 2010).

Cash-for-care schemes emphasizing autonomy and choice for recipients became a prominent approach in many recent long-term care reform efforts in Western Europe (Glendinning and Kemp 2006; Ungerson and Yeandle 2007). While long-term care systems in Central, Eastern and South-Eastern European countries are more service-oriented, they all have some tradition of care-related payments. In contrast with recent Western European developments, care-related payments in most of these countries are directed at informal caregivers, providing them with some financial recognition for the work they provide. In Hungary, for instance, payment to informal carers for care provided by them amounts to the level of the minimum pension (about €100.00 in 2006) and may be reduced to 80 per cent or increased to 130 per cent depending on the status of the person being cared for. In the Czech

Republic, earlier cash-for-care schemes have recently been replaced and substantially extended towards a care allowance paid at four different levels to those in need of care (Österle 2010).

With regard to public funding of long-term care services, very different principles apply in the health sector and the social sector. Health systems in the CSEE region are built on the social health insurance principle, even though the details of the systems are more universality-oriented in some, and more market-oriented in other countries (for overviews see Albreht *et al.* 2002; Gaál 2004; Hlavačka *et al.* 2004; Rokosová *et al.* 2005; Voncina *et al.* 2006; Waters *et al.* 2008; Vlădescu *et al.* 2008). Services for chronically ill and frail elderly people provided by the health sector include designated chronic care beds in hospitals and mobile health nursing, but the actual definition of these services and the extent of respective provisions vary widely between countries. Funding of these schemes is from the individual country's social health insurance fund and co-payments made by recipients. But the level of these co-payments is far lower than the co-payments required for similar services provided in the social care sector, which creates incentives for health-care provision rather than social care provision, where this is an option. In the social care sector, tax-based public funding is mostly social assistance-oriented, with full or virtually full public coverage limited to those cases where individuals and their families are unable to make any contribution from their regular income or assets. Public social care funding in general consists of a mix of per-bed or per-service unit remuneration and additional public subsidization (Österle 2010).

The fragmentation of existing public long-term care systems, the lack of infrastructure and the lack of resources result in generally low levels of services in these countries. Individual perceptions of availability and affordability of long-term care accord with these deficits. According to Eurobarometer 2007 data, people in CSEE countries perceive access to nursing homes and care services for dependent elderly people as being more difficult than in the EU27 average (see table 2). In six of the seven countries covered by this chapter, between 18 and 23 per cent of the interviewees perceive access to nursing homes as very easy or fairly easy, compared to 39 per cent in the EU27 average. For care services, the relevant proportion is between 24 and 33 per cent in the CSEE countries, compared to 41 per cent in the EU27 average. Also, more people in CSEE perceive services as being unaffordable, compared to the EU27 average. While just 7 per cent of the Dutch or 12 per cent of the Swedes see nursing homes as being unaffordable, it is 64 per cent in Slovenia, 58 per cent in Croatia or 52 per cent in Slovakia. These results are in line with funding schemes. While nursing home funding requires co-payments in the Netherlands or in Sweden, social assistance orientation in the study region involves substantial private contributions and, to an extent, even contributions by family members.

In a European comparative perspective, long-term care systems in CSEE may be characterized as fragmented early stage systems (Pavolini and Ranci 2008). Similar to other welfare sectors, the country-specific context but also current policy developments and policy proposals indicate that these countries will follow different routes in more comprehensively addressing the risk of long-term care. At the same time, they have a couple of major issues in common that will have to be resolved in the reform process. Three key areas will be discussed in greater detail in the following sections: (i) the fragmentation in existing welfare policies as regards the risk of long-term care dependency, in particular as between the health and social care sectors; (ii) the role of the private sector, in particular as the provider of services; and (iii) the current and future role of family care.

Fragmented Long-term Care Policies as between Health and Social Care

In the 1990s, decentralization and pluralization became major objectives driving the social policy agenda in CSEE, from the early years of transition onwards (Cerami 2006; Schubert *et al.* 2009). While the health sector (including long-term care from the health sector) remained largely centralized, responsibilities in providing and, in part, funding social services were increasingly shifted towards provincial and local levels, in particular in the Central-Eastern European region. This has further strengthened an old dividing line in services for people in need of long-term care, that between health and social sectors. While the health sector is responsible for more medically oriented institutional settings and qualified nursing care in the outpatient sector, social sector responsibilities include residential care as well as personal care, domestic help and other support programmes. The division between health care and social-care sectors, however nebulous it may sometimes be in practice, has important implications for providing and funding services.

In terms of funding, social insurance arrangements dominate the health-care sector, while tax funding and the application of social assistance principles dominate the social sector. There is budgetary pressure on both sectors, which not merely increases the financial pressure within these sectors, it also increases the incentives for actors to shift responsibilities and costs to other sectors. As a response to growing health sector expenditure, governments across the region have implemented various cost-containment approaches, not least with the attempts to reduce the number of hospital beds (Gaál 2004; Nemec and Kolisnichenko 2006). In practice, reduction of hospital beds was either achieved by closing down hospitals or hospital departments, or by transforming them into social care beds. This latter approach reduces public financial responsibilities in the health care sector, but increases pressure on the social care sector without necessarily providing an adequate infrastructure for long-term care needs. It also shifts responsibilities from the public sector to the individual, as health sector provisions are publicly funded, while social sector care pursuant to the social assistance principle involves substantial private payments (Österle 2010).

From a comparative perspective, the dividing lines between health and social care sectors are drawn quite differently across European countries. In CSEE, they tend to be quite diffuse in real life. Existing parallelism and the search for more integrated care are major concerns for governments as they pursue reform activities. At the same time, existing parallel structures and related economic incentives are major hurdles for governments in developing and implementing reforms. Following the decentralization principle, across the region, provinces and local authorities were given broader authority to develop infrastructure and provide community services. While decentralized systems can further increase diversity and fragmentation, they may also have positive effects in terms of better responding to local preferences or in terms of creating positive spill-over effects through learning from experiences in other regions (for a discussion of the situation in Southern Europe, see Costa-Font, this volume). In CSEE, however, developments in the community care sector or a diffusion of existing innovative initiatives have so far remained rather limited, because of a lack of government funding, but also because of a lack of priorities in the field of long-term care (Österle 2010).

The Emerging Welfare Mix in Long-term Care

In addition to decentralization, pluralization and privatization were major principles that accompanied the transition process in CSEE. While decentralization was a powerful factor in many ways, the process of pluralization and privatization was much slower in health care and in social care. In terms of institutional background, public sector care clearly dominates the formal provision of care in the CSEE region more than in most other European countries, which is above all a consequence of such care being covered almost exclusively by the public sector before the 1990s (Munday 2003). Private actors are still playing a minor role in residential care and in many areas of community care. There is, however, a general trend towards strengthening and incentivizing the role of private actors, in particular non-profit organizations.

Currently, in the countries being studied here, between 75 per cent (in Croatia) and almost 100 per cent of residential care beds (in Serbia) are in public institutions. Private residential care homes tend to provide smaller numbers of beds per residence compared to public sector nursing homes. The non-profit sector accounts for about one-fifth of beds in Hungary and Romania and less than 15 per cent in the other countries. All of these countries have also seen for-profit initiatives in the residential care sector, by both national and international provider organizations. The proportion of for-profit sector beds is currently more significant in South-Eastern European countries, whereas it is almost negligible in other countries (Österle 2010). With regard to social services provided in the community, the picture varies. Services provided by the health sector are predominantly in the public sector. In the social care sector, public sector services play an important role where these services have been historically more established, in urban areas in particular. Where services have been implemented more recently, non-profit organizations are playing an important role, both as initiators and as providers (Széman 2003; Dobre 2009). For Romania, for example, it is estimated that about one-third of day-care centres and about two-thirds of domiciliary care are provided by the non-profit sector (Österle 2010).

Overall, non-profit sector care in CSEE long-term care systems is a relatively new development. Some local activities have historical roots in providing services and have re-entered the social care market in the transition period. Other initiatives have developed in close cooperation with international counterparts that are providing know-how and co-funding to establish and develop infrastructure. Examples include the Red Cross or church-related organizations such as Caritas or Diakonie. But there are also grassroots initiatives, or local non-profit organizations that focused previously on other vulnerable groups in society. In South-Eastern Europe, many non-profits that have been involved in helping refugees have now shifted their focus towards other areas of social work and social assistance. Depending on where their roots lie, who their international counterparts are and what the local context is, non-profit sector initiatives are emphasizing lobbying, the provision of information or the provision of services, with the last becoming increasingly important.

Despite strong rhetoric politicians and officials use regarding pluralization and – at least in some countries – privatization, a broader welfare mix has developed rather modestly. One major source of these limitations is the often-cited relative weakness of civil society and of third-sector organizations in this region by comparison with Western Europe (e.g. Howard 2002). Though the early transition period was characterized by a 'renaissance' of civil society and significant growth in the number of non-profit organizations in many Central-Eastern European countries, these developments soon slowed down (Mansfeldová *et al.* 2004). The relative weakness of third sector developments has been characterized by various factors, including the level of civic engagement, a lack of trust in organizations, the difficult search for new relationships with the state, and, not least, the lack of income from the state (e.g. Toepler and Salamon 2003; Mansfeldová *et al.* 2004; Frič 2008; Jenei and Kuti 2008; Nemec 2008).

The limited accessibility of public funding and the regulation of underlying funding regimes are a major second reason for the limited degree of pluralization of social services and for the limited degree of expansion of such services. The lack of public co-funding, and the fact that only a very small proportion of the population can actually afford privately paid services, have hindered any larger-scale establishment of private providers. Still, some non-profit initiatives have been successful at a local level. Their development has been fostered by factors such as trust within the community, a broader willingness to support these developments via private donations, support from local or regional governments and/or financial support from international counterparts. But non-profit organizations in Romania and South-Eastern Europe have come into substantial financial trouble when financial support from international counterparts or from international assistance organizations was reduced at a time when national public authorities were unwilling or unable to make up the difference (Balogh 2008; Dobre 2009). And policies improving the financial basis for non-profit social services have often been contradictory. Many Central and Eastern European countries have introduced schemes where citizens can designate a small portion of their income tax payments for third-sector organizations. In Hungary, a '1 per cent system' was introduced in 1997 (Jenei and Kuti 2008). On the other hand, many countries have had explicit policy approaches prioritizing public provision of care over private-sector care, either in the context of accreditation or by discriminating against private providers in access to public funding (e.g.

Nemec 2008). Recent developments indicate that the pluralization rhetoric of state actors in the field of long-term care is only now being more systematically translated into policies that are intensifying the efforts to better integrate the roles of the public and the private sectors in providing care, in order to stimulate the creation of private–public partnerships and to strengthen non-profit sector contracting (Österle 2010).

Long-term Care as a Family Responsibility

In CSEE, long-term care needs in the population are mostly, and often exclusively, covered within informal networks, above all by female close family members. Under state socialism, the emphasis on participation in the workforce was the route to emancipation of women. Participation in the workforce provided access to social protection, was supported by childcare services, and led to high levels of employment. It did, however, not touch upon the division of responsibilities within families, where traditional patterns remained predominant (Pascall and Manning 2000; Pascall and Lewis 2004; Schnepf 2007). In the transition process, these traditional patterns, and the way they translated into the division of household and care work, were even reinforced. The deeply anchored values and perceptions of social family obligations in the region are also reflected in a Eurobarometer survey (European Commission 2007). Accordingly, 45 per cent of those living in the EU27 countries prefer to be cared for at home by a relative. Most Central and Eastern European countries are above this average, with peak values in Hungary (66 per cent) and in Poland (70 per cent). Also, in the Central and Eastern European region, the number of those who would prefer to move in with a family member is above the EU27 average (see table 2). According to the same survey, support for the two following arguments is stronger in these countries compared to the European average: 'Children should pay for the care of their parents if their parents' income is not sufficient' and 'Care should be provided by close relatives of the dependent person, even if that means that they have to sacrifice their career to some extent'. Significant differences between CSEE countries emerge in terms of selling the house to cover long-term care costs. This option is supported by more than half of the population in Slovenia and Croatia but by only about a quarter in most EU27 countries (see table 2 and European Commission 2007).

About 11 per cent of women and 6 per cent of men provide help and support to frail elderly or disabled people at least a couple of times a week (Anderson et al. 2009). Women are more likely to provide personal help and help in the household and it is women who work as the main carers, spending long hours on care work. A few countries in the CSEE region such as Romania and Slovakia, however, report larger shares of men being involved in long-term care work and also report longer hours of informal care work provided by men (Anderson et al. 2009; Österle 2010). Though there is no systematic assessment available, a larger unemployment rate among men, early retirement, and women migrating to Western European countries for household and care work might at least partly explain this fact. Whether this could also contribute to more gender equality in providing care, as Pascall and Lewis (2004) have suggested for the childcare sector, remains to be seen.

The extent to which families are able to perform long hours of care work is co-determined by a range of factors, not least employment patterns. In this respect, the CSEE region exhibits some particular features. A larger proportion of the population has previously given up paid work or switched to part-time employment in order to take care of an elderly parent (European Commission 2007). Compared to Western European countries, most of the CSEE countries are characterized by lower levels of employment (leaving more room for informal care activities), but also lower levels of part-time employment among those in regular employment (limiting their room for informal caregiving) (Eurostat 2009a). In line with EU employment and growth policy objectives, all of the countries are striving to increase employment levels and to increase the effective retirement age. This in turn will lower current informal long-term caregiving potential. Labour market perspectives and considerable wage differences from a subnational perspective, as well as from a European comparative perspective, have led to considerable flows of migration within countries into metropolitan areas as well as to outflows towards other European countries. This leaves many of the elderly in the more rural areas in an extremely precarious situation, all the more so as social services are often non-existent there.

The lack of a comprehensive network of services and the unequal distribution of existing services create enormous burdens on informal care arrangements. Carers, mostly women, find themselves in particularly precarious situations. Direct support for informal carers through social security coverage for informal care work, counselling and relief programmes or allowances directed at informal carers have become a more prominent policy issue in Europe very recently, even though broadly accessible policy measures remain limited in many countries (Lamura *et al.* 2008). In CSEE, care work allowances paid to informal carers are the most important and usually the only measure available to support informal carers. The level of the benefit in Hungary is oriented to the minimum pension, with the opportunity to decrease or to increase the benefit depending on the status of the person in need of care. Especially for lower-income households, the benefit can create an incentive to give up paid employment in order to be able to provide care to a close family member. It can even be an economic strategy to manage a household under extremely precarious conditions. Given the low level of the benefit and the lack of affordable additional services, it generally does not change the enormous burdens involved in informal caregiving and often prolongs a most precarious situation. Another arrangement, where women from Central and Eastern European countries commute to Western European countries as care workers, has been receiving increasing recognition. Important source countries are Slovakia and Romania, major receiving countries being Italy or Austria (e.g. Bettio *et al.* 2006; Da Roit *et al.* 2007). The specific arrangements have a multitude of implications for these care workers and for the household context in both the receiving and the source country. One aspect of this phenomenon is that income from this type of care work in both regular and irregular care markets allows these women to substantially subsidize their household budgets in their home countries. At the same time, the phenomenon often entails a rearrangement of care obligations in the home country household (Haidinger 2008).

With an existing long-term care infrastructure which is very limited and poor, with a lack of investment on new approaches, and with a rhetoric of pluralization and privatization that has not been supported by an adequate regulatory framework and adequate financial strength, the bulk of care work in the region remains with the family or in other informal arrangements. Given the above-referenced values and perceptions and the traditional division of care work, it is mainly women who provide the care. However, given the broader socio-demographic and socio-economic changes briefly addressed in the earlier sections of this chapter, the CSEE region is no exception to the fast-growing need for new approaches in addressing the risk of long-term care.

Discussion and Future Directions

This chapter has sought to explore whether countries in CSEE follow a broader European trend of major, partly path-departing long-term care reforms. The analysis has shown that in CSEE – similar to the situation in most other European countries – long-term care is a latecomer in welfare state development (Österle and Rothgang 2010). Principles such as decentralization, privatization or pluralization emphasized in social policy transformation in the CSEE region in the past twenty years had limited and delayed effects on long-term care. In recent years, debates on creating more comprehensive schemes recognizing long-term care as a social risk have intensified – even if mostly in debates confined to small expert groups. Translating these ideas into social policy reforms, however, has been hindered by fears that new welfare schemes will substantially extend public expenditure obligations, by restrictions civil society and expert groups find in bringing the issue into a broader public debate and by a failure of governments to set priorities in this sector. It is only in the Czech Republic where a newly introduced long-term care system marks a new paradigm in addressing long-term care.

Following the analysis in this chapter, current care regimes in the CSEE region can be portrayed as 'family care model' (Anttonen and Sipilä 1996) with a 'familial/individualist paradigm' (Timonen 2009). Responsibility for care is largely with families and individuals. Welfare state provision outside the health sector is mostly means-tested, limited to a relatively small proportion of the population and characterized by huge regional disparities. This current situation is challenged in manifold ways including ageing populations and increasing long-term care needs, changes in the broader socio-economic context and its implications for informal care arrangements and the financial consequences of demographic developments and policy choices. Projections of the budgetary implications of ageing European societies show the considerable financial pressure countries in Central-Eastern Europe are facing, not least in the field of long-term care (European Commission 2009b). In a pure demographic scenario, between 2007 and 2060, public expenditure on long-term care as a proportion of GDP will increase by between 149 per cent in Hungary and 221 per cent in Romania, compared to 102 per cent in the EU15 average. Changes in assumptions of disability prevalence change the extent of public expenditure increases, but do not change the sharper increases in Central-Eastern Europe. These projections, however, are based on the current long-term care policies with low levels of formal care provision in Central-Eastern Europe. When a shift from informal to formal care is taken into account, projections in the mixed home and institution scenario indicate a 129 per cent increase in public long-term expenditure in the EU15 average for the 2007–60 period. In Central-Eastern Europe, the projected increase will be 203 per cent in Slovenia, 238 per cent in the Czech Republic, 237 per cent in Slovakia, 265 per cent in Hungary and 349 per cent in Romania. In Croatia and Serbia, not included in that study, demographic pressures are smaller than in Central-Eastern Europe, but the current very low levels of formal provision will also drive public long-term care expenditure when formal care provision is extended.

Across Europe, countries are searching for a new balance of public, private and family care arrangements in order to ensure high-quality and cost-effective access to care for all citizens (European Commission 2009a; see other chapters in this book). CSEE countries largely subscribe to these objectives. But the current systems are characterized by fragmentation, huge deficits in the long-term care infrastructure and a lack of financial resources. Debates and proposals for developing a more comprehensive long-term care system have intensified only recently. In the Czech Republic these debates have led to fundamental changes in the system. The 2007 reform has built new foundations for the provision and funding of social services and emphasizes cash allowances paid to those in need of care. This marks a major turning point in the Czech long-term care system, even though it remains to be seen what further developments the implementation of the new system produces. In Slovenia, an intensive debate has led to a detailed proposal for a long-term care insurance scheme, but this has yet to be implemented. Reference to the adoption of long-term care insurance schemes can be found in all countries being studied here, even though specific proposals have not been developed to any degree approaching that in Slovenia. (For a discussion of social insurance in the field of long-term care see Barr, Rothgang, and Schut and van den Berg, this volume.) The agenda of the reform debates stresses quite similar objectives across the region: decentralization, clarification of responsibilities in funding and providing health and social care, pluralization in providing services, the development of the provision of social services in the community, the development of alternative housing arrangements, and the improvement of access and efficiency. Taken together, this recognizes the need to more comprehensively address long-term care as a social risk (European Commission 2009a; Österle 2010). If the respective policies are implemented, it would mean steps towards a care regime where states extend their financial responsibilities and where a mix of actors is engaged in service provision (Timonen 2009).

While major regulatory measures will be needed to achieve these objectives, current practices in long-term care are often driven by local or regional-level initiatives, both in the public and in the non-governmental sectors. Such practices are rooted either in traditional approaches to care for the frail elderly or in more recent developments and pilot programmes. Examples include foster care in Croatia, where people in need of care do not live with their own family, but live in another family network. In Slovenia, a pilot project in direct funding combines the need for support with the objective of achieving greater user independence by developing individual service planning. In Romania, as in the other countries being studied here, non-profit organizations have become important forerunners in developing social services in the community, in particular in those areas where such services were non-existent before. These examples of both traditional and more novel approaches have grown as a reaction to specific deficits, recognizing the particular regional or local context. They provide support that complements or serves as a substitute for traditional family care systems and create alternatives to institutionalization. Dissemination, however, remained limited, above all for budgetary reasons. Getting closer to realizing the objectives mentioned earlier in this final section will require substantial efforts on governmental levels towards developing the infrastructure in integrated and community-oriented social services, and will require an emphasis on improving availability of and access to services across countries, a focus on user needs and on quality of services, the establishment of new governance structures and sustainable public–private relationships. Governments will need to recognize long-term care as a real social risk, not just a subject for rhetorical debate, and adopt social policies which substantially increase investment in this sector.

Acknowledgements

This chapter is based on an international project on long-term care in Central and South-Eastern Europe directed by the author and undertaken in cooperation with research teams in the seven countries. Papers from the country teams are currently being reviewed for publication in an edited volume. The project was funded by ERSTE Foundation, whose support is gratefully acknowledged.

References

Alber, J. and Köhler, U. (2004), *Health and Care in an Enlarged Europe*, Luxembourg: European Foundation for the Improvement of Living and Working Conditions.

Albreht, T., Cesen, M., Hindle, D., Jakubowski, E., Kramberger, B., Petric, V., Premik, M. and Toth, M. (2002), *Slovenia: Health System Review. Health Systems in Transition*, Copenhagen: World Health Organization.

Anderson, R., Mikulič, B., Vermeylen, G., Lyly-Yrjanainen, M. and Zigante, V. (2009), *Second European Quality of Life Survey: Overview*, Luxembourg: European Foundation for the Improvement of Living and Working Conditions.

Anttonen, A. and Sipilä, J. (1996), European social care services: is it possible to identify models? *Journal of European Social Policy*, 6, 2: 87–100.

Balogh, M. (2008), The role of Romanian NGOs in the democratization process of the society after 1990. In S. Osborne (ed.), *The Third Sector in Europe: Prospects and Challenges*, London: Routledge, pp. 53–65.

Bettio, F., Simonazzi, A. and Villa, P. (2006), Change in care regimes and female migration: the 'care drain' in the Mediterranean, *Journal of European Social Policy*, 16, 3: 271–85.

Castles, F. G. and Obinger, H. (2008), Worlds, families, regimes: country clusters in European and OECD area public policy, *West European Politics*, 31, 1–2: 321–44.

Cerami, A. (2006), *Social Policy in Central and Eastern Europe: The Emergence of a New European Welfare Regime*, Berlin-Hamburg-Münster: LIT Verlag.

Da Roit, B., Le Bihan, B. and Österle, A. (2007), Long-term care policies in Italy, Austria and France: variations in cash-for-care schemes, *Social Policy & Administration*, 41, 6: 653–71.

Dobre, S. (2009), The Romanian welfare state: changing and developing. In K. Schubert, S. Hegelich and U. Bazant (eds), *The Handbook of European Welfare Systems*, London: Routledge, pp. 415–27.

Doyle, M. and Timonen, V. (2008), *Home Care for Ageing Populations: A Comparative Analysis of Domiciliary Care in Denmark, Germany and the United States*, Cheltenham: Edward Elgar.

Economic Policy Committee and European Commission (2006), *The Impact of Ageing on Public Expenditure: Projections for the EU25 Member States on Pensions, Health Care, Long-term Care, Education, and Unemployment Transfers (2004–2050)*, Special Report 1/2006, Brussels.

European Commission (2007), *Health and Long-term Care in the European Union*, Report, *Special Eurobarometer 283/Wave 67.3*, Brussels: European Commission.

European Commission (2009a), Joint report on social protection and social inclusion. Available at: http://ec.europa.eu/employment_social/spsi/docs/social_inclusion/2009/cons_pdf_cs_2009_07503_1_en.pdf (accessed 17 April 2009).

European Commission (2009b), *2009 Ageing Report: Economic and Budgetary Projections for the EU-27 Member States (2008–2060)* (provisional version), Brussels: European Commission.

Eurostat (2009a), Eurostat Database. Available at: http://epp.eurostat.ec.europa.eu. (accessed 17 April 2009).

Eurostat (2009b), Perception of health and access to health care in the EU-25 in 2007, *Statistics in Focus*, 24, Luxembourg: European Communities.

Fenger, M. (2007), Welfare regimes in Central and Eastern Europe: incorporating post-communist countries in a welfare regime typology, *Journal of Contemporary Issues in Social Sciences*, 3, 2: 1–30.

Frič, P. (2008), The uneasy partnership of the state and the third sector in the Czech Republic. In S. Osborne (ed.), *The Third Sector in Europe: Prospects and Challenges*, London: Routledge, pp. 230–55.

Gaál, P. (2004), *Hungary: Health System Review. Health Systems in Transition*, Copenhagen: World Health Organization.

Glendinning, C. and Kemp, P. (2006), *Cash and Care: Policy Challenges in the Welfare State*, Bristol: Policy Press.

Hacker, B. (2009), Hybridization instead of clustering: transformation processes of welfare policies in Central and Eastern Europe, *Social Policy & Administration*, 43, 2: 152–69.

Haidinger, B. (2008), Contingencies among households: gendered division of labour and transnational household organization – the case of Ukrainians in Austria. In H. Lutz (ed.), *Migration and Domestic Work: A European Perspective on a Global Theme*, Aldershot: Ashgate, pp. 127–42.

Hlavačka, S., Wágner, R. and Riesberg, A. (2004), *Slovakia Health System Review. Health Care Systems in Transition*, Copenhagen: World Health Organization.

Howard, M. M. (2002), The weakness of postcommunist civil society, *Journal of Democracy*, 13, 1: 157–69.

Inglot, T. (2008), *Welfare States in East Central Europe, 1919–2004*, Cambridge and New York: Cambridge University Press.

Jenei, G. and Kuti, É. (2008), The third sector and civil society. In S. Osborne (ed.), *The Third Sector in Europe: Prospects and Challenges*, London: Routledge, pp. 9–25.

Lamura, G., Döhner, H. and Kofahl, C. (eds) (2008), *Family Carers of Older People in Europe*, Münster: LIT Verlag.

McKee, M., Adany, R. and MacLehose, L. (2004), Health status and trends in candidate countries. In M. McKee, L. MacLehose and E. Nolte (eds), *Health Policy and European Union Enlargement*, Maidenhead: Open University Press, pp. 24–42.

Mansfeldová, Z., Nałęcz, S., Priller, E., and Zimmer, A. (2004), Civil society in transition: civic engagement and nonprofit organizations in Central and Eastern Europe after 1989. In A. Zimmer and E. Priller (eds), *Future of Civil Society: Making Central European Nonprofit-Organisations Work*, Wiesbaden: VS Verlag für Sozialwissenschaften, pp. 99–119.

Mete, C. (2008), *Economic Implications of Chronic Illness and Disability in Eastern Europe*, Washington, DC: World Bank.

Munday, B. (2003), *State or Civil Society? Social Care in Central and Eastern Europe*, Canterbury: European Institute of Social Services.

Munday, B. and Lane, G. (1998), *The Old and the New: Changes in Social Care in Central and Eastern Europe*, Canterbury: European Institute of Social Services.

Nemec, J. (2008), The third sector and the provision of public services in Slovakia. In S. Osborne (ed.), *The Third Sector in Europe: Prospects and Challenges*, London: Routledge, pp. 118–33.

Nemec, J. and Kolisnichenko, N. (2006), Market-based health care reforms in Central and Eastern Europe: lessons after ten years of change, *International Review of Administrative Sciences*, 72, 1: 11–26.

Österle, A. (ed.) (2010), *Long-term Care in Central and South Eastern Europe: Project Report*, Vienna.

Österle, A. and Rothgang, H. (2010), Long-term care. In F. G. Castles, S. Leibfried, J. Lewis, H. Obinger and C. Pierson (eds), *The Oxford Handbook of the Welfare State*, Oxford: Oxford University Press, pp. 405–18.

Pascall, G. and Lewis, J. (2004), Emerging gender regimes and policies for gender equality in a wider Europe, *Journal of Social Policy*, 33, 3: 373–94.

Pascall, G. and Manning, N. (2000), Gender and social policy: comparing welfare states in Central and Eastern Europe and the former Soviet Union, *Journal of European Social Policy*, 10, 3: 240–66.

Pavolini, E. and Ranci, E. (2008), Restructuring the welfare state: reforms in long-term care in Western European countries, *Journal of European Social Policy*, 18, 3: 246–59.

Ripka, V. and Mareš, M. (2009), The Czech welfare system. In K. Schubert, S. Hegelich and U. Bazant (eds), *The Handbook of European Welfare Systems*, London: Routledge, pp. 101–19.

Rokosová, M., Háva, P., Schreyögg, J. and Busse, R. (2005), *Czech Republic: Health System Review. Health Care Systems in Transition*, Copenhagen: World Health Organization.

Saxonberg, S. and Sirovatka, T. (2009), Neo-liberalism by decay? The evolution of the Czech welfare state, *Social Policy & Administration*, 43, 2: 186–203.

Schnepf, S. V. (2007), *Gender Equality in Central and Eastern Europe*, Saarbrücken: VDM.

Schubert, K., Hegelich, S. and Bazant, U. (eds) (2009), *The Handbook of European Welfare Systems*, London: Routledge.

Stubbs, P. and Zrinščak, S. (2009), Croatian social policy: the legacies of war, state-building and late Europeanization, *Social Policy & Administration*, 43, 2: 121–35.

Széman, Z. (2003), The welfare mix in Hungary as a new phenomenon, *Social Policy and Society*, 2, 2: 101–8.

Timonen, V. (2009), *Ageing Societies: A Comparative Approach*, Maidenhead: Open University Press.

Toepler, S. and Salamon, L. M. (2003), NGO development in Central and Eastern Europe: an empirical overview, *East European Quarterly*, 37, 3: 365–78.

Ungerson, C. and Yeandle, S. (2007), *Cash for Care in Developed Welfare States*, Basingstoke: Palgrave.

Vlădescu, C., Scîntee, G., Olsavszky, V., Allin, S. and Mladovsky, P. (2008), *Romania: Health System Review. Health Care Systems in Transition*, Copenhagen: World Health Organization.

Voncina, L., Jemiai, N., Merkur, S., Golna, C., Maeda, A., Chao, S. and Dzakula, A. (2006), *Croatia: Health System Review. Health Care Systems in Transition*, Copenhagen: World Health Organization.

Waters, H., Hobart, J., Forrest, C., Siemens, K., Pittman, P., Murthy, A., Vanderver, G., Anderson, G. and Morlock, L. (2008), Health insurance coverage in Central and Eastern Europe: trends and challenges, *Health Affairs*, 27, 2: 478–86.

World Health Organization (WHO) (2009), WHOSIS. Available at: www.who.int/whosis/en/ (accessed 17 April 2009).

Zatonski, W. (2007), Editorial: the East–West health gap in Europe. What are the causes? *European Journal of Public Health*, 17, 2: 121.

7

Devolution, Diversity and Welfare Reform: Long-term Care in the 'Latin Rim'

Joan Costa-Font

Introduction

The uncertain influence of governance structures on welfare-state processes and outcomes motivates inquiries into how best to define the morphology of welfare services. In the midst of a welfare retrenchment era, the importance of institutional design is particularly pertinent, especially in those areas of welfare policy where there is still a perceived need for coverage expansion, such as long-term care for the elderly in Europe.

Long-term care (LTC) includes an array of services that, in most countries, are delivered by different levels of government as well as by households. Yet, the burden of publicly financed care lies very heavily in the hands of the local governments (see Trydegård and Thorslund, this volume). Furthermore, LTC is an area of policy that straddles a largely universally funded health-care system and an underfunded system of social-care provision. Since the 1990s, nationwide schemes to finance LTC have been discussed and introduced in many European countries, including the Netherlands (see Schut and van den Berg, this volume) and the UK (see Comas-Herrera *et al.*, this volume), among others. Calls for countrywide reforms appear to be driven both by the expansion of the demand for care, especially when care shortages reach a high rung on the policy-reform ladder (Costa-Font *et al.* 2008), and by supply-side calls for structures that satisfy trade unions, regional governments and agents interested in the regulation of LTC provision and financing.

Nonetheless, the political economy of LTC reform in Europe is highly influenced by the regional and local dynamics of welfare politics, the institutional design diversity of the welfare state alongside the strength of private or independent stakeholders. Typically, the level and nature of welfare governance is often the result of path dependency and historical legacies rather than of a thoughtful examination of what would be the most efficient scale at which to provide and finance a service. Moreover, although long-term care policy is widely envisaged as a second-order political responsibility nationally, it has the potential to become a central, first-level priority of regional politics (Wincott

2006). Therefore, the influence of regional devolution of LTC policy on the dynamics of welfare reform, and the diversity of the welfare state is at the forefront of social policy debates. Decentralization can arguably give rise to regional policy processes within a country, and consequently allow for certain agendas with limited consensus nationwide to develop at a regional level (Costa-Font *et al.* forthcoming).

From all European countries, those in the so-called 'Latin Rim' (Katrougalos 1996), in particular Italy and Spain, rank high in terms of welfare fragmentation (Ferrera 1996). A typical pre-reform scenario in those countries consists of diverse and underfunded provision in the hands of local governments. Calls for reform tend to remain unattended as policy-makers – usually at central government level – succumb to the temptation of (fiscal) blame avoidance by maintaining a system where highly dispersed responsibilities in the hands of local authorities make it difficult to trace political accountability. In such a framework disagreement on how to reform the system can potentially hamper political opportunities for welfare reform nationally, by allowing veto players to block attempts of welfare reform. However, the incentives associated with the diffusion of the fiscal blame avoidance can operate in a very different way and eventually can stand in favour of welfare reform. Political opportunism can lead different levels of government to collude (sharing responsibility) or alternatively to compete on a reform. This is the case if government plans are perceived to expand coverage for welfare services that are in great demand, as was the case of LTC in Spain before the 2008 reform (Costa-Font *et al.* 2008).

This chapter pursues two goals. One is to examine the conditions of the pre-LTC reform scenario in Spain and Italy to examine the institutional mechanisms underpinning LTC reform, focusing particularly on the incentives included in regional devolution in Spain *vis-à-vis* local-level fragmentation in Italy. The second is to explore further the degree of diversity and coordination in policy design and welfare service supply resulting from devolution.

The structure of the chapter is as follows. The first section is devoted to the current understanding of devolution, reform and welfare state diversity. The next one presents the long-term care systems in the two countries. Then the diversity and differentiation in policy design and in supply is reported, followed by a discussion on the reform inception. The last section summarizes the main findings and contains a discussion on policy implications.

Background

Devolution and reform

Absence of welfare reform is frequently justified by the existence of path dependence. That is, if institutions are 'locked in' to a certain path, reform becomes costly to implement even when the objective conditions to change exist (Liebowitz and Margolis 1995; Kay 2005). In regionally devolved welfare states, path dependence has at least two opposite effects. An old political economy approach would suggest that welfare-state federalism (or devolution seen as a form of 'informal federalism') impedes welfare-state development by introducing veto points to welfare reform. Pierson (1996) more generally argues that reform opportunities improve when the number of decision-makers declines; the fewer the institutional obstacles, the higher the likelihood of reform.

On the other hand, new approaches to political economy acknowledge that federalism tends to act as a reform catalyst in areas where there is widespread support for reform, and perception of the need for reform is widespread. More importantly, political incentives for credit-claiming through LTC reform become especially relevant under an *ageing electorate*. In such a setting, welfare decentralization could become a reform catalyst via new dynamics[1] and sources of legitimacy (Braun *et al.* 2002). Decentralization, it has been argued, can help to diffuse the financial blame by transferring fiscal responsibilities to other layers of government (Banting 2005). Hence, devolution can offer an opportunity to bypass the stylized fact whereby reforms tend to be paralysed when their fiscal burden affects a broad group of the electorate (e.g. in the form of tax rises, use of regionally decentralized resources, etc.). A common reaction to overcome path dependence by central level incumbents is to collude with the opposition to avoid taking the blame in the event of a reform backfiring. In other words, to pass the fiscal blame down to the lowest possible level of government, or to diffuse it by involving a multitude of intermediate decision-makers (Weaver 1986).[2]

In addition to blame shifting to other levels of goverment, reforms in LTC tend to come with limited public subsidization. This is a common device to shift the load of the reform to the users themselves by reducing the intensity and increasing the cost sharing of the care covered rather than the number of entitlements (Simonazzi 2009). Hence, incumbents can still claim credit for the reform, and more generally their political support for dependent elderly people in society remains intact. However, they do so by passing on a significant share of the welfare costs to the public through cost-sharing mechanisms. Hence, the diffusion of the financial blame encompasses blame-sharing with other levels of government and when possible the opposition along with users themselves.

Devolution and diversity

Probably the most common objection to welfare state devolution is based on the idea that it leads to diversity and threatens uniformity (Redwood 1999). Some other criticisms of devolved welfare systems lie in that it might inhibit welfare development (Lovering 1999) – by exacerbating region-specific lobbying; similarly, devolution is argued to hinder government efficiency due to a lack of management capacity, or a lack of local legitimacy and transparency in some regions (Heald *et al.* 1998). However, proponents of devolution argue that as a governance model it can give rise to competition (or cooperation) among regional governments and spill-over effects, especially when a neighbouring government's performance is taken as a yardstick to evaluate regional welfare policy (Salmon 1987). Devolution also responds best to local preferences when heterogeneity in regional preferences makes the 'strategy of equality' (or uniformity) socially undesirable (Costa-Font *et al.* 2006). However, possibly the most powerful argument for devolution is that it acts as a 'laboratory for experimentation' if regional social care regulation and region-specific policies are developed, some of which draw upon learning from the experiences of other regions. Finally, the main argument put forward in this chapter is that a regionally organized welfare system can help rationalize regional political representation (of locally scattered services) alongside enhancing the interaction between central and regional welfare-policy interests increasing political accountability. A devolved form of administration by giving rise to new political agency ralationships, motivates regional incumbents to pursue reform strategies so as to legitimize their policies. Similarly, it can help to reduce institutional fragmentation by setting up policies that coordinate welfare within their regional territories. To date, there has been little research on whether devolution as a type of institutional design actually prevents welfare development in the area of long-term care, and particularly on whether differences arise in the dynamics of decentralization or federalism (Morel 2004).

Long-term Care in the 'Latin Rim'

This section attempts to describe the key characteristics of the organization of LTC in the Latin Rim countries examined. Possibly the most important feature of Latin Rim models of LTC lies in its privatization of LTC, which has traditionally been informally provided within the household (Costa-Font and Vilalta 2006; Costa-Font and Rovira 2008), and reliance on the public sector that is mostly seen as a last resort. Traditionally, in-kind support is scarce and locally managed, while central government intervention tends to take the form of cash allowances (Italy) or tax reliefs (Spain). Significantly, responsibilities for LTC are highly devolved to regional governments and/or local authorities. Yet, even though Italy and Spain share similar patterns, they exhibit significant differences in LTC organization and funding alongside the model of regional devolution.

The Spanish model is based on a central government that coordinates and provides a basic regulatory framework[3] while the actual policies and regulation are designed by the regional governments. Regional governments are responsible for the organization of health care and the coordination of social services which are managed by the local authorities. Both regional governments and local authorities are financed by their own taxes alongside tax revenues that are vertically assigned through block grants allocated on an unadjusted capitation system. Similarly, in Italy the central government defines the basic framework, and the regulation of health policy is designed by the regions, whereas social care (with the exception of a few regional guidelines) is designed by individual municipalities.[4] There are two main publicly funded home-care services: integrated domiciliary care (*assistenza domiciliare integrata*) and home help. Home help is delivered by municipalities and home health care is provided by the local health authorities (*Azienda Unità Sanitaria Locale*). In both Italy and Spain, nationwide

Figure 1

Percentage of the elderly (65+) receiving the 'companion payment'
(*indennità di accompagnamento*)

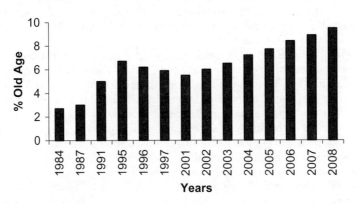

Source: ISTAT, several years.

coordination plans have been carried out over the years, but with no significant effect.

In a pre-reform scenario, the most important policy in place refers to a nationwide allowance known as the 'companion payment' (*CP*; *indennità di accompagnamento*) in Italy. This is a needs-based allowance paid irrespective of the claimant's financial conditions and financed by the central government through taxation. The payment enables the old-age dependent person to buy commercial services or it can be passed on to caregiving relatives and is completely detached from the provision of in-kind services (Gori and Da Roit 2007). It was introduced in 1980 for non-elderly disabled people and was extended to the over-65s in 1988. In 1984, some 2.7 per cent of the elderly received the CP and this percentage rose to 5.0 at the beginning of the 1990s (1991) and increased to 9.5 in 2008 (see figure 1). This sharp growth was due to four main factors: (a) augmented needs: there was a huge increase in the percentage of people over 80, and a decrease in the availability of informal care was under way; (b) low provision of in-kind services: the number of home-care users increased, but not enough, and most users received only a few hours care a week; (c) the system of incentives: the eligibility criteria set at national level are quite vague and local health authorities – led by the regional governments – are motivated to interpret them generously as they face a huge demand, and state funding for the *indennità* is open-ended; and (d) a surge of previously deterred applicants. No equivalent scheme existed in Spain.

Fragmentation and Diversity

Next, the dynamics of devolution and institutional interactions in both Italy and Spain are examined, questioning how they influenced the fragmentation and diversity in their welfare services. Devolution is traditionally associated with diversity because it allows governments to experiment and follow an incremental reform process, whereby marginal reforms lead to more important ones until eventually a paradigm shift takes place (Hall 1993). This is particularly the case in Spain, where regional devolution has acted as an institutional device to adjust institutional designs and policies to regional preferences (Costa-Font and Rico 2006).

In Spain, differences in priorities between regional programmes explain different policies throughout the territory. From the very beginning of the devolution process, various regional governments created agencies to coordinate health and social care in order to provide an integral service to their citizens. For example, Catalonia, Castile-Leon and Cantabria have prioritized the integration of health and social care, while other regions, such as the Basque Country and Galicia focus on the development of personal social care. The regional government of Valencia governed by the conservatives implemented an innovative nursing-home voucher scheme, whose main objectives were to increase users' choice and reduce waiting lists (Tortosa and Granell 2002). Finally, Andalusia (1999), Madrid (1998) and the Canary Islands (1997) have designed regional specific social service plans to coordinate services in its regions. More generally, the decentralization process in Spain has led to a growing regional diversity in policy-making alongside further coordination within regions, by setting regional targets and regional specific institutions, that are diffused to other regions.

Similarly, in Italy, the impact of decentralization on policy innovation has been notable at the local level; however, coordination within regions to reduce fragmentation has not been a priority. In the absence of a national reform, many regional governments introduced far-reaching reforms, though these were mostly the regions that already had the highest coverage of services and the most advanced policy environment, such as Emilia-Romagna, Lombardy, Tuscany and Veneto. Diversity is reflected in the balance between different services. In some regions the priority has been community care (e.g. Emilia-Romagna) whereas others have chosen residential care (e.g. Lombardy). Recently, debate has centred on how to guarantee the same formal care provision for all elderly people with the same needs within a region. Three policy strategies are currently under way: (a) introducing entitlement packages at an individual level for all the elderly people living in the region with the same needs (Tuscany); (b) equalizing the economic resources for care provision available to local authorities in all the sub-areas of a region, through an adjusted capitation system for the elderly (Emilia-Romagna); (c) not introducing a policy to assure equity in care (Lombardy). Another key issue in the recent debate was whether or not to introduce users' freedom of choice. In 2003 Lombardy introduced a voucher system for most community-care services (*assistenza domiciliare integrata*) which enables users to choose one service provider from among different competing offers. The other regions did not set up free-choice systems. More than four years after its inception, the voucher system was under question, according to the Lombardy administration's own sources (Regione Lombardia 2008). Hence, limited diffusion has taken place, as well as its reform constraints.

Reform: Institutional and Political Determinants

In identifying the sources of reform, it is necessary to both understand the demand for long-term care coverage. Generally, demand for the development of public long-term care coverage comes mainly from lower- and middle-class households who are struggling to bear the costs of paying for the care of elderly dependants informally within the household (Costa-Font *et al.* 2008). The incorporation of female workers into the labour market curtails the availability of caregivers within the household, and social changes impedes the reproduction of the traditional social model. In addition the modernization of perceptions of independence and care availability increase the demand coming from elderly dependants themselves. In Spain, this has led to a situation where the demand for nursing-home places exceeds supply. By the mid-1980s, around 100,000 older people were on waiting lists for a room in a public nursing home.

Public decision-makers, however, are faced with cost-containment pressures and the general commitment to fiscal stability and austerity affecting all European Union member states. During the 1990s, cost-containment pressures impeded the development of long-term care services in both Italy and Spain. However, in 2005, in the middle of an expansionary business cycle and after an unexpected electoral victory, the Spanish socialist government finally decided to make a move towards the implementation of long-term care reform, free-riding on drafts by previous governments that had not managed to attain sufficient support from trade unions, the financial sector, regional governments and other stakeholders. Previous governments had also met with other restraints, including the view that long-term care should be largely funded by some form of life-savings – indicating the resilience of an inheritance culture based on intergenerational bequests – and, partly as a result of the latter, a general unwillingness to redistribute wealth.

The Spanish case

With the exception of an allowance for the elderly disabled in 1982, very limited reform in the area of long-term care took place during the 1980s. In that period there were several attempts to reform the system but, given that all regions set up their own social service regulation between 1982 and 1992, central-level regulation was ineffective, appearing as meaningless and legally unconstitutional. During the period of conservative government from 1996 to 2003, opposition, mainly from Andalusia and the trade unions along with lack of political visibility and limited consensus, stood as the main impediments to reform, and so it had limited success. However, the political scenario shifted after 2003 when the socialist party recovered power.

In 2006, after several years of discussion and debate – with draft proposals dating back to 1999 – the Spanish parliament approved the introduction of a 'national system of long-term care' for dependent people of any age. It came into effect in January 2007, though it will not be totally operative until

2015. It was formally defined as a 'universal' system, in which access to long-term care is described as a 'personal right'. This programme covered a 'basic package' intended to be accessible by anyone, anywhere in Spain, and complementary packages provided and financed by the regional governments, the contents of which depended on their own choices. It was agreed that funding would be shared between central government and the autonomous regions. Dependent individuals were expected to co-pay in accordance with their income; those who could afford to pay for long-term care were to contribute up to 90 per cent of the total costs. On average, cost-sharing was estimated to account for between 30 and 35 per cent of total costs and no tax was associated with the funding of the system. Care provision was both public and private, and home help was the key service. The reform's definition of dependency was in line with that of other countries such as Germany.[5] However, in Spain, the theory and practice of the reform have been markedly different. The reform was envisaged on the basis of an optimistic growth scenario and, due to the recession, the speed of application has not been what was expected. The inception of the system drew heavily upon the existing social-security surplus, which accounted for as much as 1 per cent of GDP in 2005 but which subsequently disappeared due to the economic downturn.

The process initiated in Spain resembled the reform in Germany, where the *Land* governments proposed long-term care reforms (Campbell and Morgan 2005), although, unlike Germany, the role of the Senate was quite restricted and was replaced by an inoperative system of territorial representation. Another shared feature of the Spanish and German reforms was political disagreement within the right wing on how to push forward the reform, although the conservatives in Spain failed to find enough common ground among stakeholders to sustain a reform. Finally, agreement was reached by convincing those opposed to the reform of the need for rationalization of long-term care provision. In both countries right- and left-wing parties worked together to promote the reform. In Spain, the socialist government saw long-term care as their most important social package, and opportunistically used their political influence in key regional governments, such as Catalonia and Galicia, to push through an agreement on funding: one-third was to be financed by funds allocated by regional governments and one-third by individual users through cost-sharing schemes.

The political conditions for reform in Spain were extremely favourable. The reform met ideal conditions on three key aspects: timing (economic expansion), cross-party coalition-building (blame avoidance) and ways of framing and packaging policy to guarantee public acceptance (high social demand). Furthermore, the reform took place when the newly elected socialist government was very strong and worked in coalition with regional parties in Catalonia and Galicia. The reform not only required individual support – registered as high in opinion polls – but also commitment by key region states to refrain from vetoing the reform and to participate in its funding. The fact that a socialist central government coincided with a coalition of socialists and left-wing parties in the regional governments of Catalonia and Galicia minimized the chances of a veto by the regional governments. There was some opposition to the reform from Basque nationalists in Navarre and the Basque Country, because the reform constituted a central government ruling on devolved fiscal responsibilities. Hence, they saw the reform as overriding transferred responsibilities in a way that was not envisaged in the bilateral fiscal agreements made between the Basque and Spanish governments. In Catalonia, the opposition party (Catalan nationalists) opposed the system on similar grounds, but this was mainly a strategic move, designed to express its ideological and opportunistic rejection of a newly created left-wing coalition government in Catalonia.

At a national level, the conservative opposition did not oppose the reform immediately, thus diffusing potential fiscal costs of the reform even further. This was because the reform had been initiated by the opposition party when in government (previous drafts dated back to 1999). However, once the reform was passed, the regional governments of Madrid and Valencia, run by the conservative opposition, opposed it by delaying implementation and drawing up region-specific regulations. As shown in figure 2, the two region states with the lowest percentage of elderly people benefiting from the reform are key region states governed by the conservative opposition namely, Madrid and Valencia.[6] Thus, political opportunism on the side of the governing socialist party and coalition-building with advocates of decentraliza-

Figure 2

Percentage of the elderly receiving subsidized care after the 2007 regulation in Spain (2009)

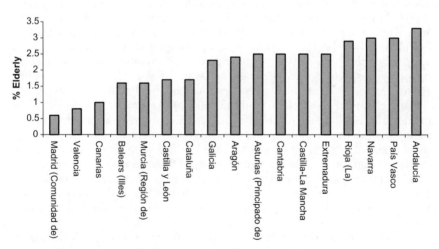

*Regional governments on the lower axis, from left to right: Madrid (Community of); Valencia; Canary Islands; Balearic Islands; Murcia (Region of); Castile and Leon; Catalonia; Galicia; Aragon; Asturias (Principality of); Cantabria; Castile-la Mancha; Extremadura; la Rioja; Navarre; the Basque Country; Andalusia.
Source: IMSERSO, several years.

tion opened the door to the reform, although it could not prevent some vertical competition from regions governed by the opposition, to delay its implementation.

The Italian case

National long-term care reform has been under discussion for several decades in Italy, but no government has seriously worked to introduce it. The Italian institutional model of governance and politics stands at the core of this question. Typically, the only welfare issues that generally attain political support in Italy are those concerning pensions, health care and the labour market. Very little support is given to issues concerning long-term care, poverty, unemployment or childcare. However, one stark difference with Spain (and Germany) is that in Italy regional governments have been unable to push the national government into passing long-term care reforms. Instead, their strategies aim at obtaining as much funding as possible for their regional health care service.

In Italy reform unavoidably requires the modification of the 'companion payment' (*indennità di accompagnamento*) for severely disabled people, now affecting 9.5 per cent of the population, especially in the poorest areas of the country – mostly in the South – where it is sometimes unofficially used as a measure to support low-income families, filling the gap left by the lack of unemployment benefits and income-support schemes in Italy. Furthermore, about 10 per cent of the users (deaf and blind persons) receive a higher payment of about €700 a month. All of these factors make reforming the companion payment a difficult political task. Furthermore, overcoming the historical inertia in place implies garnering sufficient support to weaken the traditional veto points blocking reform, especially in a country such as Italy where governments are usually politically quite weak (Kazepov 2008).

Public debate on the need for national long-term care reform began in 1997, when the centre-left government led by Romano Prodi set up a commission of experts, named *Commissione Onofri* after its chair, the economist Paolo Onofri, to design an overall reform of the Italian welfare system, including long-term care. The Commission made several proposals, including one for national long-term care reform, but these proposals were never implemented. Since then various politicians and trade unions have made proposals for a national reform, all of which share the following aims: (a) to increase public expenditure devoted to long-term care; (b) to increase the provision of in-kind services; and (c) to reduce the enormous inter-regional differences in the amount of public care provision. Nevertheless, the goal of national long-term care reform failed to gain attention and support in the Italian policy arena.

Unlike in Spain, where reform took place in a period of economic expansion, and where a central level public budget expansion could be ring-fenced, in Italy tight control of public outlays and limited representation of the frail elderly impeded credit-claiming and blame diffusion. Furthermore, regional governments in Italy have rarely exerted strong pressures on the agenda at the national level to reform long-term care. A nationwide reform would have two looser groups namely, the deaf and blind people who are currently privileged with a relatively generous allowance alongside the poor and unemployed population of some deprived areas. With respect to national long-term care policy-making, the 20 Italian regions did not manage to function as one single actor in the national political arena. Instead, the representatives of the 20 regions were quite effective in forcing the government to increase funding for health care and in preventing it from cutting expenditure when it planned to do so. More importantly, unlike Spain, regions failed to pressure the government into introducing the long-awaited national reform of long-term care.

Discussion

Reform of the provision and financing of long-term care for the elderly is a common feature of welfare developments in Europe. This chapter draws upon the experiences of two 'Latin Rim' countries, namely Italy and Spain to examine how devolution influences welfare reform. I contend that welfare coverage reform in Italy and Spain has followed different institutional trajectories despite similar departure conditions in the early 1980s – heavy fragmentation and reliance on means-tested cash payments. The findings indicate that in Spain, progressive decentralization of social care to the newly created regional governments, gave rise to welfare reform. In Italy, however, failure to rationalize social care can be partially attributed to the difficulties in credit-claiming, since social care for the elderly is not an area of responsibility that has traditionally attracted significant political attention both at national and regional level. Regional decentralization of LTC was not an institutional reform welcomed by regional incumbents unless it encompassed an expansion of regional funding.

This chapter's findings indicate that although the two Latin Rim countries departed from similar starting points they exhibit heterogeneous institutional and political trajectories alongside cross-country socio-demographic compositions. The Spanish example is consistent with a process of regional-level rescaling of long-term care responsibilities[7] as part of a strategy of democratization and modernization that covers health, education and social care. Regional devolution in Spain seems not to have increased fragmentation and to have enabled, to an extent, the consolidation of a nationwide entitlement to long-term care services for the dependent elderly. This contrasts with the Italian case where, as mentioned, we find inertia[8] and limited entitlement to in-kind care, where the absence of political opportunity for blame avoidance has impeded reform, especially when regions do not wish to bear the costs of an unfunded social care system. As a result, social care has remained a local-government responsibility and not been coordinated with regionally provided health care.

Political explanations are not negligible in the Spanish case. Indeed, the fact that in Spain similar political interests coincided at central and regional government levels and that the reform had the support of the opposition (which initiated it) had the effect of diffusing responsibilities, increasing opportunities for blame avoidance, and thus minimizing the risk of a reform veto. Furthermore, although the Spanish reform was seen as an invasion of regionalized social policy responsibilities by the Basque national-ists and Catalan nationalists, the fact that a coalition of socialists and left-wing parties in Catalonia and Galicia coincided with a socialist central government created the political conditions for reform by diffusing political blame region-ally. The conservative opposition initially backed the government on the reform, but simultaneously used the two key regional governments run by them at the time (Madrid and Valencia) to effectively block its implementation by failing to coordinate with central government plans. However, tensions remain as to differences in the scrutiny of dependency claims, the central state contribution and especially the final contribution of individuals themselves (SAAD 2009).

Acknowledgement

The author is grateful to Bent Greve, Valentina Ziganti and Cristiano Gori for suggestions and clarifications. The author is fully responsible for the content and the usual disclaimer applies.

Notes

1. Decentralization is argued to produce invasions of policy space occupied by one level of government by another level, forcing reactive changes that, in turn, induce further change (Anton 1997).
2. The capacity to do this will depend on risk adjustment processes. For instance, the cooperative federalist structure in Germany provides incentives to shift fiscal burdens back to central government level (Campbell and Morgan 2005).
3. Responsibilities for health and social care have been unified into a single ministry and the Institute of the Elderly and Social Services (IMSERSO) – a central agency run by the Spanish Ministry of Labour and Social Affairs – contributes to define, coordinate and monitor LTC policies at national level. Up until 2008 the main instruments used at central government level were the National Gerontological Plans (*Planes gerontologicos*); however, they had very little effect.
4. At the national level there is a Secretary of State for Employment, Health and Social Affairs, in charge of both health care and social care, while within each region there is one minister in charge of health and another responsible for social care.
5. Potential users are assessed at local level, using the same instrument throughout the whole country. If they are deemed eligible, they are then grouped into three levels of dependency.
6. The regional government of Madrid even contested the reform legislation in a constitutional court, arguing that regulation on social care is a decentralized responsibility.
7. Indeed, reforms in federal states such as the United States indicate that the responsibility for long-term care of frail elderly people has shifted from local to regional governments (Ogden and Adams 2008). Similar processes can be identi-fied in other countries, especially those that have regionalized their welfare system as a result of processes of political and fiscal decentralization.
8. As argued later, the fact that health and social care coincide at the same govern-ment level has enabled some coordination to occur in Spain, while lack of coordi-nation is the norm in Italy.

References

Anton, T. J. (1997), New federalism and intergovernmental fiscal relationships: the implications for health policy, *Journal of Health Politics, Policy, and Law*, 22, 3: 691–720.

Banting, K. (2005), Canada: nation-building in a federal welfare state. In H. Obinger, S. Leibfried, and F. G. Castles (eds), *Federalism and the Welfare State: New World and European Experiences*, Cambridge: Cambridge University Press, pp. 89–137.

Braun, D., Bullinger, A.-B. and Walti, S. (2002), The influence of federalism on fiscal policy making, *European Journal of Political Research*, 41, 1: 115–45.

Campbell, A. L. and Morgan, K. J. (2005), Federalism and the politics of old age in Germany and the United States, *Comparative Political Studies*, 38, 8: 887–914.

Costa-Font, J. and Font-Vilalta, M. (2006), The limits to the design of long-term care insurance schemes: the Spanish experience in comparative research, *International Social Security Review*, 59, 4: 91–110.

Costa-Font, J. and Rico, A. (2006), Vertical competition in the Spanish National Health System, *Public Choice*, 128: 477–98.

Costa-Font, J. and Rovira, J. (2008), Who is willing to pay for long-term care insurance in Catalonia? *Health Policy*, 86, 1: 72–84.

Costa-Font, J., Elvira, O. and Mascarilla, O. (2006), Means testing and the heterogeneity of housing assets: funding long-term care in Spain, *Social Policy & Administration*, 40, 5: 543–59.

Costa-Font, J., Garcia, A. and Font-Vilalta, M. (2008), Relative income and attitudes towards long-term care financing, *Geneva Papers of Risk and Insurance*, 33, 4: 673–93.

Costa-Font, J., Salvador, L., Alouso, S., Cabases, J. and McDaid, D. (forthcoming), Tackling neglect and mental health care reform in a devolved system of welfare governance, *Journal of Social Policy*.

Ferrera, M. (1996), The 'Southern model' of welfare in Social Europe, *Journal of European Social Policy*, 6, 1: 17–37.

Gori, C. and Da Roit, B. (2007), The commodification of care – the Italian way. In C. Ungerson, and S. Yeandle, *Cash for Care in Developed Welfare States*, Basingstoke: Palgrave, pp. 60–80.

Hall, P. (1993), Policy paradigms, social learning and the state, *Comparative Politics*, 25: 275–96.

Heald, D., Geaughan, N. and Robb, C. (1998), Financial arrangements for UK devolution, *Regional and Federal Studies*, 8: 23–52.

Katrougalos, G. S. (1996), The South European welfare model: the Greek welfare state, in search of an identity, *Journal of European Social Policy*, 6: 39–60.

Kay, A. (2005), A critique of the use of path dependency in policy studies, *Public Administration*, 83: 553–71.

Kazepov, Y. (2008), The subsidiarization of social policies: actors, processes and impacts. Some reflections on the Italian case from a European perspective, *European Societies*, 10, 2: 247–73.

Liebowitz, S. and Margolis, S. (1995), Path dependence, lock-in and history, *Journal of Law, Economics and Organization*, 11: 205–26.

Lovering, J. (1999), Theory led by policy: the inadequacies of the 'new regionalism', *International Journal of Urban and Regional Research*, 23: 379–95.

Morel, N. (2004), Providing coverage against new social risks in Bismarckian welfare states: the case of long-term care. Paper presented at l'ISA RC19 annual conference, Paris, 2–4 September.

Ogden, L. L. and Adams, K. (2008), Poorhouse to warehouse: institutional long-term care in the United States, *Publius: The Journal of Federalism*, 39, 1: 138–63.

Pierson, P. (1996), The new politics of the welfare state, *World Politics*, 48, 2: 143–79.

Redwood, J. (1999), *The Death of Britain*, Basingstoke: Macmillan.

Regione Lombardia (2008), *Bilancio sociale dell'Assessorato alla famiglia e delle politiche sociali*, Milan: Lombardy Region.

SAAD (2009), Informe final del grupo de expertos para la evaluación del desarrollo y efectiva aplicación de la ley 39/2006 14 de diciembre de promoción de la autonomía personal y atención a las personas en situación de dependencia, Ministry of Labour and Social Affairs, 22 October, Madrid.

Salmon, P. (1987), Decentralisation as an inceptive scheme, *Oxford Review of Economic Policy*, 3: 24–43.

Simonazzi, A. (2009), Care regimes and national employment, *Cambridge Journal of Economics*, 33: 211–32.

Tortosa, M. A. and Granell, R. (2002), Nursing home vouchers in Spain: the Valencian experience, *Ageing and Society*, 22: 669–87.

Weaver, R. K. (1986), The politics of blame avoidance, *Journal of Public Policy*, 6, 4: 371–98.

Wincott, D. (2006), Social policy and social citizenship: Britain's welfare states, *Publius: The Journal of Federalism*, 36, 2: 169–88.

8

One Uniform Welfare State or a Multitude of Welfare Municipalities? The Evolution of Local Variation in Swedish Elder Care

Gun-Britt Trydegård and Mats Thorslund

Introduction

In the Nordic welfare states, including Sweden, there is a potential tension between two main social policy principles: universalism and local autonomy. A welfare policy of universalistic nature is established at the national level, but implementation of the policy is a responsibility of highly independent local authorities, 'welfare municipalities' (Kröger 1997).

A decentralized authority model is likely to give rise to increasing local disparities, while greater centralization generally leads to more uniformity (Powell and Boyne 2001). Burau and Kröger (2004: 795) have emphasized the balancing act between the principles of universalism and local autonomy and termed it 'decentralized universalism'. They underline that this is a continuing process and find periods of both centralization and decentralization during the postwar era. In the Nordic countries, increasing decentralization characterized the 1990s, while a growing concern about regional inequality seems to have given rise to more central control in the early 2000s (Bergmark and Minas 2007; Kröger 2009).

In this chapter, we aim to study the evolution of the balance between universal, centralized and local, decentralized principles in Swedish welfare services, using elder care as a case study. In the light of ongoing changes and reductions at the average national level, we follow up previous studies and explore the provision of home-based as well as residential care to the oldest persons (80 years and over) at the local level, in all Swedish municipalities, over time. How has the variation between municipalities evolved over the last decades – is it constant, has it increased or have the lately observed centralization tendencies led to decreased variation? How strongly related is the local elder-care coverage of today to the coverage of previous years? In other words, is there a path dependency at the municipal level, indicating that local social policies exist, relatively independent of a national attempt at steering?

Universalism and local autonomy: an ongoing dilemma

In the social policy literature the Nordic countries are placed in a special welfare state model, 'a universal citizenship-based model with a high level of generosity' (Greve 2004: 158). In Esping-Andersen's terminology they represent the Social Democratic welfare state regime, in which all citizens are incorporated under one universal system. Social policy is comprehensive, embracing an extensive range of social needs and includes the entire population, regardless of income and position in the labour market (Esping-Andersen and Korpi 1987). The Nordic welfare system is based on a high degree of universalism and equality (Kautto *et al.* 1999; Anttonen 2002). Another main principle is to minimize dependence on families, with the state taking responsibility for the care of children, the aged, and disabled persons (Esping-Andersen 1990). Thus, the Nordic welfare state is not only a 'social insurance state' but also a 'social service state' (Anttonen 1990). In recent years, scholars have pointed out that the similarities between the Nordic countries are no longer so pronounced. For instance, in a study of elder-care development between 1980 and 2000, Rauch (2008) finds that Denmark has kept its universality, while Sweden has developed a more selective system (see also Szebehely 2005a).

Even though the concept of universalism is frequently used to characterize this welfare state regime, it is often loosely used and defined differently (Kröger *et al.* 2003). Sometimes universalism is defined by its antithesis/ antipode: it is not selective, not only for the poor, not means-tested, not based on individuals' contributions (Anttonen 2002; Rauch 2008). There seems, however, to be consensus about some characteristics of universalism, suggested by Anttonen (2002): benefits and services should be based in legislation, tax-financed, available to and used by all citizens in need, irrespective of income and place of residence – services should be equal across the nation (see also Kröger *et al.* 2003; Greve 2004; Rauch 2008). According to Anttonen, universalism can be stronger or weaker, depending on how many of the suggested criteria are fulfilled.

One other characteristic trait in the Scandinavian welfare model is that welfare services, such as childcare, elder care and disability care, are organized in a much decentralized system. The main responsibility for the social services rests with highly autonomous local governments. 'Welfare municipalities' is a concept which has been used to underline the significant role of independent municipalities in the distribution of social services in the Nordic countries (Kröger 1997; Trydegård and Thorslund 2000). The dilemma or tension between the national welfare state principles of universalism, generosity and equality on the one side, and the varying local implementation of the policy on the other, has been stressed by numerous researchers, and many studies have demonstrated large local variation in different forms of social services (see e.g. Kröger 1997; Palme *et al.* 2002; Lewin *et al.* 2008; Rauch 2008).

Whether the local diversity in service provision is a sign of geographical inequality and territorial injustice has been debated in the literature (Boyne and Powell 1991), and the question of a spatial division of welfare has been raised in several studies from different countries and different policy areas (for a broad overview, see Powell and Boyne 2001). Some researchers have stressed the advantages of decentralized welfare, arguing that geographical variations may be regarded as evidence of successful responsiveness to needs in the local population (Powell and Boyne 2001: 186; Savla *et al.* 2008), and that the empowerment of local government in the Social Democratic welfare states has been a condition to make this type of welfare state possible (Sellers and Lidström 2007). On the other hand, strong municipal autonomy and varying access to services can also be seen as a threat to a universal and equitable social service system (Rauch 2008). In a universal welfare state citizens might expect that equal access to and equivalent standard of care and services should not depend on one's residential location; otherwise the citizens' confidence in the system and their willingness to pay taxes is undermined (Trydegård and Thorslund 2000; Bergmark and Minas 2007).

The central–local balance in Swedish elder care

According to the Swedish constitution, local governments enjoy great autonomy and can decide independently on their own affairs – locally elected politicians make all major policy decisions in respect of their areas of responsibility, and the municipal council and committees establish goals and guidelines for local government operations. They also approve the budget, set the local income tax rate, decide on eligibility criteria and the size of the fees charged for local services (Bergmark and Minas 2007). The 290 Swedish municipalities vary greatly in population and in character, from big cities to sparsely populated rural areas. In terms of population size, the municipalities vary between 2,500 and 810,000 inhabitants, with a median of 15,500 (Statistics Sweden 2008).

The central government's main instruments of control are legislation, state subsidies and supervision through central agencies, and within the field of elder care these are rather weak. The *legislation*, the Social Services Act from 1982, is in the nature of a goal-oriented framework law without detailed regulations, leaving it to the local authorities to decide on the means to reach the goal. The individual is entitled to assistance on a 'reasonable level of living', if 'his/her needs cannot be met in any other way', wordings which can be interpreted in different ways by different local authorities. The needs assessment is made by a local social worker (care manager) who is delegated by the social welfare committee to decide on what kind of, and how much, help and assistance the elderly person will receive, whether in the form of home help services or residential care, and also the income-adjusted fee to be paid. Most municipalities have elaborated local guidelines which have turned out to have a strong impact on the care managers' assessments and decisions (Larsson 2005). Also, the local supply of services and care has proved to influence the decisions and the assistance the elderly persons receive (Lindelöf and Rönnbäck 2004; Dunér and Nordström 2009). The *state subsidies* changed in the mid-1990s from ear-marked to block grants, calculated on the basis of a municipality's revenues and estimated expenses, and taking into account structural factors such as the age, living conditions, and socio-economic status of the local population. This new system did away with state control of how the money was used, thereby giving the municipalities greater freedom – and potentially also leading to greater variation among municipalities (Bergmark and Minas 2007). The *state supervision* through the National Board of Health and Welfare (NBHW) and through national authorities on the regional level is of a consultative nature, but has been intensified and stressed in recent years. NBHW has for instance been mandated by the government to publish annual open comparisons of municipalities' elder-care operations for benchmarking purposes.

Thus, the development from the 1980s to the mid-1990s was mainly characterized by decentralizing trends. Framework laws were introduced, state subsidies became general, and in many welfare areas responsibility was transferred from central or regional to local levels, for instance all long-term care for older people as well as services and support to physically and mentally disabled persons. By contrast, from the second half of the 1990s there have been centralizing trends through a more detailed and compulsory legislation for persons with severe disabilities, a maximum-fee reform to cap user fees in elder care, and also some targeted government grants for specific measures which the government wants to prioritize, most recently the clients' freedom of choice in elder care (Bergmark and Minas 2007). In this volume, the same tendency of decentralized long-term care is reported also from England, Spain and Italy, and South-Eastern Europe (see Comas-Herrera *et al.*, Costa-Font, and Österle, this volume).

One crucial question is how the central–local balance of power influences the municipal variations in supply, accessibility and quality of services and care. In the 1990s large local variations in the distribution of elder care were reported from the Nordic countries (see e.g. Berg *et al.* 1993; Sundström and Thorslund 1994; Boll Hansen and Platz 1995; Naess and Waerness 1996; Daatland 1997). Trydegård and Thorslund (2000) revealed a large diversity in coverage rate for home help as well as residential care in the Swedish municipalities in the mid-1990s. The variations were to a very small extent explained by differences in the population or municipality structure, or by local government economy and politics, and variation also increased during the 1990s. However, there was an obvious 'path dependency' at the local level; even though all municipalities reduced their home help coverage, the majority of the municipalities maintained a rather stable local pathway in relation to the average development in Sweden. Municipalities seemed to have developed local social policies in their services to older persons in accordance with local traditions and historical continuity (Trydegård 2000). Considering the tendencies of increased centralization which have been reported lately, the question arises whether these tendencies have resulted in less variation between municipalities in the provision of elder care.

Material and Methods

For the empirical analyses in this chapter, official statistics on municipal elder-care services in Sweden were used. For aggregated data on the national level we also used a compilation of comparable data made by the Ministry of

Health and Social Affairs (2002). Our study concerns the two main services to older people: home help in ordinary housing and residential care of a different kind (in service houses/sheltered housing, old-age homes, nursing homes, group dwellings, etc.). The Swedish municipalities also offer complementary services, such as meals-on-wheels, day care, short-term care, but as these are of minor extent and often combined with either home help or special housing, we concentrate on the two most widespread services.

To be able to compare between municipalities of different population size we use the coverage rate, i.e. the percentage of municipal residents of a certain age receiving services at a given time. We have chosen to study the oldest age group, 80 years and over, because in this age group we find the frailest elderly persons whose needs are difficult to ignore. Living alone is also most common in the oldest age group, a condition that makes elderly people more dependent on public services (Larsson and Thorslund 2002).

Comparable data at the municipal level concerning services to persons aged 80 years and over were available from 1993 up to 2006. The year 1993 is a good starting point for comparison as this was the first year after an extensive community care reform in 1992 (the ÄDEL reform) whereby responsibility for all kinds of long-term care for elderly persons was shifted from the county councils to the municipalities (NBHW 2008). After 2006 there are no comparable data – from the year 2007 statistics on social services were gathered at the individual client level, which makes comparisons to earlier years impossible (NBHW 2009). Data on the national level are available for a wider time span, in which the 1992 shift of responsible authority for long-term care is adjusted for (Ministry for Health and Social Affairs 2002). Here we use 1982 as the starting point, the year when the Social Services Act was introduced and home help services were mandated by law.

Generosity of Coverage: A Sign of Universalism

As stated above, the universal welfare state is characterized by a high level of generosity in the distribution of assistance, services and care (Greve 2004). High coverage rates indicate that services are widespread and available to persons in need, while low coverage rates might be a sign of a strict allocation and a more selective model of welfare. To explore how universal Swedish elder care is from this perspective we studied the coverage rates of the two main forms of public elder care in Sweden, home help services and residential care – separately and taken together – over the past 25 years.

Figure 1 shows that public care for the oldest persons in the population in Sweden has decreased substantially during the past two to three decades. In 1982, about 57 per cent of those aged 80 years and over received either home help or residential care, compared to 37 per cent in 2006. In the 1980s the decrease was extensive, while in the 1990s it was more moderate, but still declining. From the year 2000 there is again a rather steep decrease. The substantial reduction over time cannot be explained by a corresponding improvement in health and functional ability among the oldest in the population (Larsson 2006). Instead, studies have shown that needs assessments have become much stricter, leaving persons with less extensive needs for assistance outside the public system (Thorslund 2004; Szebehely 2005b; Thorslund and Silverstein 2009). In this respect, elder care has become more selective and less universal.

Figure 1 also shows that the home help distribution line is intertwined with that of residential care, indicating that the two services can compensate for each other. When residential care coverage declines in the early 1990s, home help coverage increases, and when a larger proportion of elderly people receives residential care, as in the late 1990s, the home help coverage drops. The Swedish home help system has the capacity to offer intensive home care, also around the clock, and can therefore be an alternative when residential care supply is insufficient. However, the steep decline in residential care from the year 2000 has not fully been compensated by a rise in coverage of home help.

The two graph lines are both descending, but the paths are not consistently straight – both have their ups and downs. Residential care coverage shows a considerable decrease from 1988 but the path changes after 1992, probably as an effect of temporary state subsidies in that period for the construction and rebuilding of special housing units for elderly and disabled persons, which resulted in the building of almost 30,000 new or modernized rooms or flats (Szebehely 1999; Parliamentary Auditors 2001). The most remarkable trend, however, is the decline in coverage of residential care starting in the year 2000. One reason behind this decrease is that many municipalities closed down

Figure 1

Coverage rates of home help and residential care for older persons (80 years and over) in Sweden 1982–2006

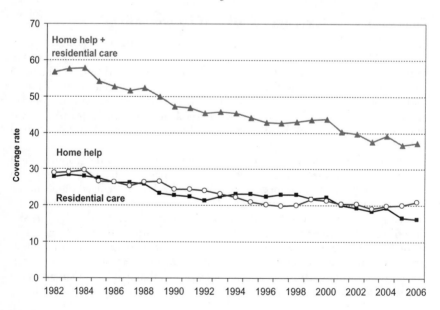

most of their so-called service houses (sheltered housing) in their capacity as 'special housing' and converted them into 'senior housing'. In senior housing the care-needing inhabitants are defined as home-help recipients, and the municipality has less responsibility for their potential health-care needs (Government Report 2008).

The decrease of home help coverage started in the mid-1980s and continued till 2002, when there was a trend break. However, the number of home help hours has increased (not shown in the figure), because resources have increasingly been concentrated on fewer and more care-demanding elderly persons – home help services as well as residential care have become intensified (NBHW 2008). This development should be seen in the light of the interdependence between two welfare programmes, social care and health care. First, an organizational reform in the elder-care system in 1992 (the ÄDEL reform) transferred responsibility for *all* long-term care for elderly people (also health care) from the county councils to local authorities. There was also a financial incentive included in the reform. The municipalities were obliged to arrange community care and support for so-called 'bed blockers', i.e. hospital patients who were medically ready for discharge, but still in need of assistance and care. Otherwise the municipalities had to pay a penalty-fee for each day the patient 'blocked the bed'. A second factor behind the intensified municipal elder care is the considerable cut-backs in the health-care sector during the financial crisis of the 1990s in Sweden. The number of hospital beds and the length of stays in hospital were drastically reduced – both were almost cut in half – and patients were sent home 'quicker and sicker' (Palme *et al.* 2002). Elderly persons with extensive needs, who were previously helped within the health-care system, nowadays take an increasing proportion of the municipal elder-care resources, in residential as well as in home-based care.

Home help services have changed and put the main emphasis on personal care and home nursing care, also round-the-clock, whereas domestic services such as cleaning, laundry, shopping and social commitments such as 'walks and talks' are increasingly put outside the municipal undertakings. Studies also show a class-related help pattern when older persons try to replace or supplement public home care. People with higher education tend to replace insufficient municipal home care with services bought on the market, while elderly persons with less education more often receive assistance from family members outside the household (Szebehely and Trydegård 2007).

To sum up the national level, Swedish elder care no longer appears to be characterized by strong universalism, either in the sense of being broad, widespread and generous, or in the sense of being equally distributed to all citizens in need.

Local Variation over Time

From a national perspective, the recent development of Swedish elder care appears rather complex. As a consequence of a centrally decided reform (the ÄDEL reform), resulting in decentralization of authority, as well as the financial crisis on national, regional and local levels, municipalities have been

Figure 2

The Swedish municipalities by the coverage rate of residential care and home help to older people 80 years and over, 1993 and 2006. Vertical and horizontal unbroken lines indicating national average

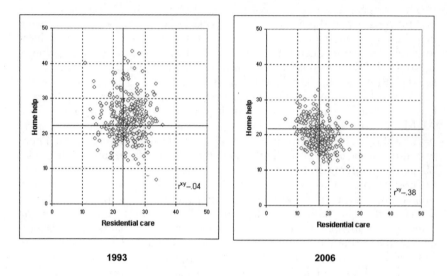

1993   2006

forced to adjust their elder care activities. What have been the consequences of this at the local level? Does the strong local autonomy lead to municipalities acting differently when struck by financial constraints? Were the widespread local variations, which were reported from the early 1990s, constant, or have they diminished or enlarged? To explore this, we used two scatter-diagrams, illustrating the care distributions of 1993 and 2006, and showing the position of all Swedish municipalities according to their coverage of residential care and home help, respectively. Such a diagram shows the dispersion of, and the relation between, the two care services. The mean coverage rates at the national level were also displayed in the figures as vertical and horizontal unbroken lines.

The two diagrams in figure 2 describe rather different distributions. In 1993 the dispersion was extensive: home help coverage ranged roughly between 13 and 40 per cent ($s = 6.0$), and residential care between 13 and 33 per cent ($s = 4.6$). The correlation between the two services was almost zero (Pearson's $r = -0.04$) at this point of time. The national average was about 23 per cent in both care services. In 2006 the picture was rather different. Besides the national averages having decreased substantially – in residential care to 16.2 per cent and to a minor extent in home help services to 20.9 per cent – the variation has diminished: in 2006, home help ranged roughly between 12 and 30 per cent ($s = 3.8$) and residential care between 10 and 25 per cent ($s = 3.6$). There is now also an apparent negative correlation between the two care services (Pearson's $r = -0.38$).

To conclude, the two diagrams in figure 2 indicate different trends in the distribution of elder care in Sweden between 1993 and 2006. First, the access to residential care has been reduced substantially, actually by one-fourth for elderly persons aged 80 years and over, while the access to home help is only slightly diminished, thanks to the rise in recent years (as illustrated in figure 1). Second, the municipal diversity in coverage has diminished, most markedly in home help services. The municipalities now describe a more compact cluster, gathered around the national average. The local variation, which was reported to be extensive in the 1990s, is now apparently reduced. Third, the relation between the two services has also changed. In the mid-1990s municipalities did not tend to substitute low access to residential care by high access to home help services, or vice versa, which they seem to do to a much higher extent in the mid-2000s. Fourth, we can also see another sign of weaker universalism in the Swedish elder-care system: when we compare the municipalities' position in relation to the national average, we find that in 2006 there are considerably fewer municipalities in the 'generous' upper right square, where municipalities with high coverage of both services are positioned. Moreover, if we had placed the average lines from 1993 in the 2006 graph, actually only one municipality would have had its position in this 'much-of-both-square'.

The scatter diagrams in figure 2 illustrate the local variation at two points of time. In order to quantify the continuing development in this respect we use a relative measure, *coefficient of variation*, i.e. the standard variation relative to the mean. A high coefficient of variation reflects a high degree of disparity or heterogeneity, and vice versa; a lower coefficient of variation indicates greater homogeneity. In figure 3 we account for the relative variation in home help services, residential care and the two services taken together, for each year between 1993 and 2006.

When we look at the two elder-care services taken together, we can see that the relative variation between municipalities lies at nearly the same level during the 1990s, but from the year 2001 there is a downward tendency. Home help services are fluctuating the most; the variation is extensive in the 1990s (which has been demonstrated in several studies, see above), but from the year 2001 it is descending, indicating less disparity between municipalities in recent years. By contrast, the variation in residential care is comparably low in the 1990s and ascending from the year 2001, so the local variation is now larger in residential care than in home help services.

Do Local Social Policies Exist in the 2000s?

A previous study (Trydegård 2000) indicated that Swedish municipalities developed local social policies in elder-care services according to local traditions and historical continuity – in the 1980s and early 1990s there seemed to be a rather strong 'path dependency'. One question raised in this chapter is whether the local continuity still remains. One way of exploring this is to study how current home help and residential care coverage are related to the coverage of previous years. We calculated the correlation (Pearson's *r*)

Figure 3

The relative dispersion (coefficient of variation) of home help and residential care for older persons in the Swedish municipalities 1993–2006

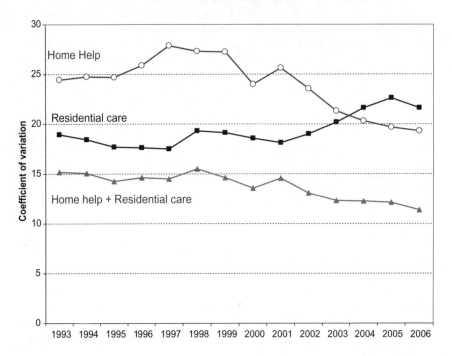

between the coverage rates of all municipalities in 2006 and those in each preceding year back to 1993. In figure 4 we account for the correlation after 1, 5, 9 and 13 years.

Two tendencies are obvious at first sight. One is that the correlation values turn out to be on different levels. As might be expected, correlation is stronger in residential care than in home help services. The latter do not require investments in physical buildings and can therefore more easily be adjusted to current care needs and demands as well as to the actual political and economic situation in the municipality. In other words, there is a stronger local path dependency in residential care than in home help services. The second tendency is that the shorter the time interval is, the stronger the correlation. After one year the correlation is substantial, 0.94 in residential care and 0.83 in home help services, corresponding to an explained variance of 88 and 69 per cent, respectively. Then it drops rather steeply: after five years to 0.52 and 0.41 respectively (corresponding to 27 and 17 per cent explained variance), and after 13 years to 0.26 and 0.13 (7 and 2 per cent explained variance). In the study mentioned above (Trydegård 2000), home help coverage five years earlier explained more than 50 per cent of the variation across municipalities

Figure 4

Correlation between coverage rates 2006 and 1, 5, 9 and 13 years earlier for home help services and residential care of older persons, 80 years and over

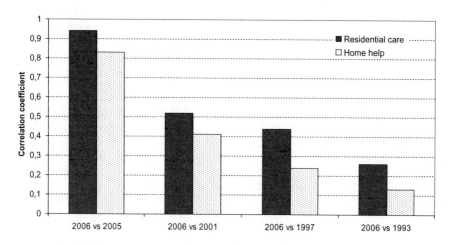

in the 1980s and 22 per cent in the 1990s. Home help services appear to be more volatile and flexible in the mid-2000s than they were during the decades before.

New Tendencies Emerging: A Concluding Discussion

With this chapter we intend to make an empirical contribution to the discussion about two contrasting principles apparent in the Nordic welfare state model – universalism and local autonomy – using Swedish elder care as a case study. We contrast our present findings to previous studies. These suggested that the extensive local variation in the service distribution made the concept of diverse welfare municipalities more adequate in describing elder-care services in Sweden, and that the universalistic principle of equal access to services for all citizens across the nation was threatened by this local variation. The 1990s were characterized by a high degree of decentralization as far as elder care was concerned – the central state influences in the form of legislation, state subsidies and control were weakened, and municipalities appeared to develop their own local policies. Local autonomy was strong at the cost of universal access to services for all care-needing citizens, irrespective of residence.

A predominant impression from our present exploration is that many aspects have changed during the first decade of the new millennium, resulting in a rather complex and inconsistent pattern. On the one hand, universalism in terms of a generous and equal distribution is weaker. The coverage of the two care services added together has decreased by one-fifth since the year 2000. Moreover, there are obviously fewer municipalities which can be designated as generous in the supply of both care services. This is consistent with the fact that the whole public sector in Sweden has been subject to financial restraint since the crisis in the 1990s, and the municipalities have been forced to carry out severe cut-backs at the same time as the elderly population has increased substantially. Services have become more selective and resources have been concentrated to persons with the greatest needs. A class-related pattern has also been visible when older persons try to replace or supplement insufficient public care. On the other hand, universalism seems stronger, considering the earlier large local variation. Municipalities are very much adjusting to the national average, and in the year 2006 they had become less diverse and more uniform in their distribution of care services. Further, the earlier reported geographical dispersion appears to have been reduced.

In the case of home help services, the municipalities still vary in coverage, but since the year 2001 there has been a larger homogeneity – the cross-municipal variation has decreased, in both absolute and relative terms. The municipalities appear to be increasingly adjusting to the national average. Our findings in this respect are in line with studies in which individual and municipal-level data were combined (Davey *et al.* 2006; Savla *et al.* 2008). Analysing the distribution of home help services to persons aged 65 years and older in Sweden in 2002–3, they concluded that a large part of the variation in coverage reflected differences regarding levels of need within the elderly populations and that home help services were distributed 'unequally, but equitably' (Davey *et al.* 2006: 40).

The coverage of residential care shows a divergent pattern – the relative dispersion has increased since the year 2001, and is now larger than in the home help services. To understand this phenomenon we must consider the development at the national level and take into account the remarkable decline in coverage rate which occurred at the start of the 2000s. The coverage decreased by one-fourth – which was not fully compensated by increased home help. The Swedish municipalities have acted in varying ways in this matter; about half of them have reduced their supply of residential care by more than 10 per cent, but of these municipalities only half have increased the access to home help correspondingly (NBHW 2005). It appears that the municipal variation is not so easily levelled out when it comes to residential care, which might be explained by the presence of physical buildings.

In the chapter we also tried to assess the municipal continuity indicating the presence of local social policies, by means of the correlation between the coverage rates of 2006 and the preceding years back to 1993. These calculations, too, showed a change compared to corresponding studies of home help coverage in the municipalities in the 1970s, 1980s and 1990s (Trydegård 2000), which revealed a strong inertia during the 1970s and 1980s, and a weaker but not unimportant one in the 1990s. Our recent study demonstrated a stronger stability in residential care than in home help services (again, probably explained by the physical buildings) but the relation to the past was weaker than before. After five years the earlier coverage of home help explained markedly less of the variation, compared to the previous study. The municipal traditions appear to have faded out, and local social policies are not as explicit as before; instead, the municipalities seem to adopt a more 'streamlined' and uniform elder care, adjusting increasingly to the national average. The development today is characterized more by centralization tendencies while the earlier very strong decentralized pattern has become weaker.

Yet another remaining question is how these rather remarkable changes in welfare distribution can be explained. What are the reasons for the strong local autonomy of Swedish municipalities not having had the same impact on the distribution of elder-care services today as it had in the 1990s? The steering instruments of the central state have not been altered in any essential way during the last decades – the national policy is unchanged, the legislation has not been revised and the state grants are still of a general nature, leaving the municipalities freedom to decide on their priorities. The state, however, also executes supervision and control through the National Board of Health and Welfare and through the regional state authorities, the county administrative boards, and the Parliamentary Auditors. In annual reports on the situation in elder care and in other publications the authorities have called attention to the variation between municipalities as regards prioritization, coverage, and costs (see e.g. Parliamentary Auditors 2001; NBHW 2008, and annual reports). The authorities have also stressed the importance of systematic and equivalent needs assessments in elder care, and decided on qualification requirements for elder-care managers, which might have an equalizing effect on the distribution of services (NBHW 2006). In recent years, the authorities have also placed emphasis on municipal comparisons and benchmarking of quality indicators in elder care, which might be another way of levelling out local variation. This kind of softer regulation has been reported to influence both the provision and the quality of services and care in the health-care sector (Bejerot and Hasselbladh 2008), and it is reasonable to think that the same phenomenon also might occur in social elder-care services. Chapters in this volume indicate similar tendencies in other European countries: suggestions from central authorities of more uniform and controlled needs assessments in order to ensure clients an equal treatment (see Comas-Herrera, and Schut and van den Berg, this volume), and publication of quality inspections of elder-care units for benchmarking purposes (see Rothgang, this volume).

To conclude: our empirical findings from the first decade of the 2000s indicate a somewhat disparate development of the balancing act between universal, centralized versus local, decentralized principles in Swedish elder care. The coverage of home help and residential care has become less generous, a sign of weaker universalism. On the other hand, the decentralization tendencies have decreased, the earlier reported geographical disparity appears to have been reduced, and the municipalities are increasingly adjusting to the national average, indicating a stronger centralization. Also, the earlier strong local path dependency has faded out and therefore the concepts 'welfare municipality' and 'local social policy' appear to be less accurate than heretofore when describing the Swedish model of elder care.

Acknowledgements

This study was supported by two research programmes financed by the Swedish council for working life and social research, 'Ageing and diversity:

living conditions and health in Sweden's elderly population' and 'Transformations of care: living the consequences of changing public policies'. The authors thank Professor Gabrielle Meagher, Sydney University, for valuable advice in the course of writing, and an anonymous reviewer for constructive comments on an earlier draft of the chapter.

References

Anttonen, A. (1990), The feminization of the Scandinavian welfare state. The welfare state in transition: from the social insurance state towards the social service state. In L. Simonen (ed.), *Finnish Debates on Women's Studies*, Tampere: University of Tampere, Research Institute for Social Science, pp. 3–49.

Anttonen, A. (2002), Universalism and social policy: a Nordic-feminist revaluation, *NORA*, 10, 2: 71–80.

Bejerot, E. and Hasselbladh, H. (2008), Det nya regleringslandskapet [The new regulating landscape]. In H. Hasselbladh, E. Bejerot and R. Å. Gustafsson (eds), *Bortom New Public Management: institutionell transformation i svensk sjukvård* [Beyond New Public Management: institutional transformation in Swedish health care], Lund: Academia adacta, pp. 107–19.

Berg, S., Branch, L. G., Doyle, A. and Sundström, G. (1993), Local variations in old-age care in the welfare state: the case of Sweden, *Health Policy*, 24, 175–86.

Bergmark, Å. and Minas, R. (2007), Decentraliserad välfärd eller medborgerliga rättigheter? Om omfördelning av makt och ansvar mellan stat och kommun [Decentralized welfare or citizenship rights? On redistribution of power and responsibility between nation state and local government], *Socialvetenskaplig Tidskrift*, 14, 2–3: 220–41.

Boll Hansen, E. and Platz, M. (1995), *Kommunernes tilbud til eldre: kommenteret tabelsamling* [Offers from municipalities to elderly people: a commented table collection], Copenhagen: AKF Forlaget.

Boyne, G. and Powell, M. (1991), Territorial justice: a review of theory and evidence, *Political Geography Quarterly*, 10, 3: 263–81.

Burau, V. and Kröger, T. (2004), The local and the national in community care: exploring policy and politics in Finland and Britain, *Social Policy & Administration*, 38, 7: 793–810.

Daatland, S. O. (1997), Welfare policies for older people in transition? Emerging trends and comparative perspectives, *Scandinavian Journal of Social Welfare*, 6: 153–61.

Davey, A., Johansson, L., Malmberg, B. and Sundström, G. (2006), Unequal but equitable: an analysis of variations in old-age care in Sweden, *European Journal of Ageing*, 3: 34–40.

Dunér, A. and Nordström, M. (2009), Gör om mig – en studie om klientifieringsprocessen i äldreomsorgen [Remake me – a study of the clientization process in elder care], *Socionomens Forskningssupplement*, 25: 44–53.

Esping-Andersen, G. (1990), *The Three Worlds of Welfare Capitalism*, Cambridge: Polity Press.

Esping-Andersen, G. and Korpi, W. (1987), From poor relief to institutional welfare states: the development of Scandinavian social policy. In R. Eriksson, E. J. Hansen, S. Ringen and H. Uusitalo (eds), *The Scandinavian Model: Welfare States and Welfare Research*, New York: M. E. Sharpe, pp. 39–74.

Government Report 2008:113, *Bo bra hela livet* [Good housing all through life], Slutbetänkande från äldreboendedelegationen [Final report from the elder housing committee].

Greve, B. (2004), Denmark: universal or not so universal welfare state, *Social Policy & Administration*, 38, 2: 156–69.

Kautto, M., Heikkilä, M., Hvinden, B., Marklund, S. and Ploug, N. (1999), The Nordic welfare states in the 1990s. In M. Kautto *et al.* (eds), *Nordic Social Policy: Changing Welfare States*, London: Routledge, pp. 1–18.

Kröger, T. (1997), Local government in Scandinavia: autonomous or integrated into the welfare state? In J. Sipilä (ed.), *Social Care Services: The Key to the Scandinavian Welfare Model*, Aldershot: Avebury, pp. 95–108.

Kröger, T. (2009), The Nordic welfare municipality: old and new variations in care policies. Conference presentation, International Conference 'Local Social Policy', Hamburg, 24–25 April.

Kröger, T., Anttonen, A. and Sipilä, J. (2003), Social care in Finland: stronger and weaker forms of universalism. In A. Anttonen, J. Baldock and J. Sipilä (eds), *The Young, the Old and the State: Social Care Systems in Five Industrial Nations*, Cheltenham: Edward Elgar, pp. 25–54.

Larsson, K. (2005), *Hemtjänsten och de äldres behov över tid* [Home help services and older persons' needs over time], Stockholm: National Board of Health and Welfare (NBHW).

Larsson, K. (2006), Hemtjänst och anhörigvård [Public home help and informal care]. In *Äldres levnadsförhållanden: Arbete, ekonomi, hälsa och sociala nätverk 1980–2003* [Elderly persons' living conditions: work, economy, health and social networks], Stockholm: Statistics Sweden, pp. 421–34.

Larsson, K. and Thorslund, M. (2002), Does gender matter? Differences in pattern of informal support and formal services in a Swedish urban population, *Research on Aging*, 24: 308–37.

Lewin, B., Westin, L. and Lewin, L. (2008), Needs and ambitions in Swedish disability care, *Scandinavian Journal of Disability Research*, 10, 4: 237–57.

Lindelöf, M. and Rönnbäck, E. (2004), Att fördela bistånd: om handläggningsprocessen inom äldreomsorgen [Distributing assistance to the elderly: the case handling process within elder care]. PhD thesis, Umeå University.

Ministry of Health and Social Affairs (2002), *Välfärdsfakta social: En sammanställning av fakta/nyckeltal inom välfärdsområdet* [Social welfare facts: a compilation of facts/ratios in welfare], Stockholm: Ministry of Health and Social Affairs.

Naess, S. and Waerness, K. (1996), *Bedre omsorg? Kommunal eldreomsorg 1980–1995* [Better care? Municipal old-age care 1980–1995], Bergen: SEFOS.

NBHW (2005), *Vård och omsorg om äldre: Lägesrapporten 2004* [Care for the elderly: report of the situation 2004], Stockholm: NBHW.

NBHW (2006), *Socialt arbete med äldre: Förslag till kompetensbeskrivning för handläggare inom äldreomsorg* [Social work with elderly persons: suggestion of qualification requirements for elder-care managers], Stockholm: NBHW.

NBHW (2008), *Development in the Care for the Elderly in Sweden 2007*, Stockholm: NBHW.

NBHW (2009), *Äldre: vård och omsorg den 30 juni 2008* [Care of elderly persons 30 June 2008], Annual Statistics, Stockholm: NBHW.

Palme, J. *et al.* (2002), *Welfare in Sweden: The Balance Sheet for the 1990s*, Final report of the Welfare Commission, Stockholm: Ministry of Health and Social Affairs.

Parliamentary Auditors (2001), *Nationella mål i kommunernas äldreomsorg* [National goals for municipal elder care], Rapport 2001/02:15.

Powell, M. and Boyne, G. (2001), The spatial strategy of equality and the spatial division of welfare, *Social Policy & Administration*, 35, 2: 181–94.

Rauch, D. (2008), Central versus local service regulation: accounting for diverging old-age care developments in Sweden and Denmark, 1980–2000, *Social Policy & Administration*, 42, 3: 267–87.

Savla, J., Davey, A., Sundström, G., Zarit, S. H. and Malmberg, B. (2008), Home help services in Sweden: responsiveness to changing demographics and needs, *European Journal of Ageing*, 5: 47–55.

Sellers, J. M. and Lidström, A. (2007), Decentralization, local government, and the welfare state, *Governance: An International Journal of Policy, Administration, and Institutions*, 20, 4: 609–32.

Statistics Sweden (2008), *Befolkningsstatistiken* [Population statistics].

Sundström, G. and Thorslund, M. (1994), Sweden: ideals and realities of old-age care in the welfare state. In D. G. Gill and S. R. Ingman (eds), *Eldercare, Distributive Justice, and the Welfare State: Retrenchment or Expansion*, Albany: State University of New York Press, pp. 25–42.

Szebehely, M. (1999), Caring for frail older persons in Scandinavia: the impact of moving borders between traditional institutions and care at home. OECD Social policy studies, unpublished report.

Szebehely, M. (2005a), Äldreomsorger i Norden: Verksamheter, forskning och statistik [Elder care services in the Nordic countries: activities, research and statistics]. In M. Szebehely (ed.), *Äldreomsorgsforskning i Norden: En översikt* [Nordic elder care research: an overview], TemaNord 2005:508, Copenhagen: Nordic Council of Ministers, pp. 21–51.

Szebehely, M. (2005b), Care as employment and welfare provision: child care and elder care in Sweden at the dawn of the 21st century. In H. M. Dahl and T. Rask Eriksen (eds), *Dilemmas of Care in the Nordic Welfare State*, Aldershot: Ashgate, pp. 80–98.

Szebehely, M. and Trydegård, G. (2007), Omsorgstjänster för äldre och funktionshindrade: skilda villkor, skilda trender? [Care services for elderly and disabled persons: different conditions, different trends?], *Socialvetenskaplig Tidskrift*, 14, 2–3: 197–219.

Thorslund, M. (2004), The Swedish model: current trends and challenges for the future. In M. Knapp, A. Netten, J.-L. Fernandez and D. Challis (eds), *Matching Resources and Needs*, Aldershot: Ashgate, pp. 119–28.

Thorslund, M. and Silverstein, M. (2009), Care for older adults in the welfare state: theories, policies and realities. In V. Bengtson, D. Gans, N. Putney and M. Silverstein (eds), *Handbook of Theories of Aging*, New York: Springer, pp. 629–39.

Trydegård, G. (2000), Tradition, change and variation: past and present trends in public old-age care. PhD thesis, Stockholm University.

Trydegård, G. and Thorslund, M. (2000), Inequality in the welfare state? Local variation in old-age care – the case of Sweden, *International Journal of Social Welfare*, 10: 174–84.

9

Reforming Long-term Care in Portugal: Dealing with the Multidimensional Character of Quality

Silvina Santana

Introduction

Until the 1970s, direct families of people with disability or chronic disease were the primary providers of long-term care, a common situation across the world with few variations. Formal long-term care was rare and generally confined to institutional care for the poor (World Health Organization 2007). Since then, the situation has changed significantly, due to much discussed socio-demographic and epidemiological factors. One of the consequences is a growing demand for home-based long-term care that might translate differently in high-, middle- and low-income countries but which is always part of major changes going on in health and social care systems.

This chapter provides an overview of the informal and institutional setting of long-term care (LTC) in Portugal and focuses on service quality, discussing this issue alongside broader problems related to the organization of LTC in the country. We argue that in the actual situation of ongoing reform of LTC in Portugal, quality assessment and management are critical actions that must be planned and implemented alongside major efforts being made. It is therefore fundamental to research how this crucial facet is being handled and perceived by the several stakeholders.

In order to properly frame the analysis, we will use a working definition of long-term care as care provided to people with physical or mental handicaps and the frail and elderly in need of support and help in their daily activities. This might include health care. However, most activities do not belong to the medical domain but to the social field and probably demand little technical knowledge and capability but a lot of social expertise. Quality is understood here as a multidimensional concept, entailing objective but also subjective aspects, that might be partially evaluated using well established and recognized standards, models and methodologies, but is always connected to each user's needs, expectations, motivations, perception, experience and capacity to learn and to the effort and resources required to provide a suitable level of service from the perspective of all the stakeholders involved.

The study is based on analysis of documents and data provided by organizations such as the INE (National Institute of Statistics), the RNCCI (National Network for Long-term Integrated Care), the Ministry of Employment and Social Solidarity (*Ministério do Trabalho e da Solidariedade Social*) and the Eurobarometer, among others.

The chapter starts by providing an overview of quality in LTC and of its informal and institutional setting in Portugal, including historical and socio-cultural roots, development and current structure and functioning. It then goes deeper into analysis of the main providers, discussing structural, organizational, quality and financing aspects of a very complex situation that is currently evolving at a very fast pace, in adapting to Portuguese society's new needs in the social care network and the recent introduction of what is designated as a third level of care, the National Network of Long-term Integrated Care (*Rede Nacional de Cuidados Continuados Integrados* – RNCCI), created by law. After that, we present results of the first self-assessments these bodies have made of the quality and suitability of services provided from the users' point of view. In order to better understand the attitudes, needs and expectations of Portuguese citizens regarding long-term care and care of the elderly and the extent to which they are being fulfilled, we then analyse the results of a survey conducted by the Eurobarometer between 25 May and 30 June 2007. Finally, we reframe the discussion and conclude the chapter by setting some lines for future work in this area.

Quality as a Multidimensional Concept

The OECD has defined long-term care as 'a cross-cutting policy issue that brings together a range of services for persons who are dependent on help with basic activities of daily living over an extended period of time' (OECD 2005: 10). Components include basic medical services, home nursing, rehabilitation, social care, housing and a wide range of services that ranges from transport, meals and laundry to instrumental activities of daily life and occupational and empowerment activities. It is important to recognize that different definitions of LTC coexist within the European Union (EC 2008) as the exact meaning of 'long' changes from country to country. It seems that the functions and services provided are more important for the definition than the length of the period of care (Driest 2006).

Quality is under increasing scrutiny in all activities and sectors related to the provision of health and social care, because of the need to respond to customer needs, expectations and concerns in a cost-effective manner that can guarantee the sustainability of systems. This holds particularly true for an ageing Europe with a tradition of systems partially or totally funded by the state, and Portugal is no exception.

With the increasing spread of long-term care (European Commission 2003) and recent reports of 'poor conditions, neglect and abuse, and medical errors in long-term care facilities' (Sorenson 2007a: 1), its quality has become an urgent matter for local, regional, and national policy-makers (European Commission 2003). Ensuring quality in the organization and delivery of health care and long-term care is now a key policy concern in all member states of the

European Community (European Commission 2003). Hopefully, quality measurement will help towards regulation in setting standards, monitoring performance and empowering citizens to make better choices.

Due to the characteristics of long-term care, namely its goals, interactions, types of public involved and their respective needs, and the environments in which it takes place, quality of care encompasses social and health facets of care, many disciplines and specialities and diverse actors, and emphasizes the value of good integration. In this context, the multidimensional character of quality becomes evident and the challenge entailed in planning, implementation and evaluation also becomes clear.

The object of assessment ranges from clinical expertise and treatment to diverse groups of services provided in different settings to assist patients with a variety of limitations. Measures include structure, process or outcome indicators, and often a mix of them is used. Objective and subjective aspects are generally included and data are collected at patient and provider levels, either through standardized instruments or more ad hoc initiatives.

Concerning health care, many attempts are being made by governments all over the world to implement quality management in public health systems but experience has been mixed (Satia 1999; European Commission 2003; Breckenkamp et al. 2007). The United States is the origin of most initiatives and reforms of long-term care quality measurement and reporting, an effort that dates from the mid-1980s, when a committee of the Institute of Medicine began studying the quality of care in nursing homes. One of the recommendations issued was mandating comprehensive assessment able to provide a uniform basis for establishing a nursing home resident's plan of care – the minimum data set (MDS) (Mor 2005; Rahman and Applebaum 2009). To monitor the quality of care for patients of home health agencies, OASIS (Outcome and Assessment Information Set) was developed in the 1990s while OSCAR (On-line Survey and Certification and Reporting System) was established for Medicare and Medicaid certified health facilities such as hospices, rehabilitation centres and nursing homes (Sorenson 2007b). OSCAR data may be used to connect MDS with facility-related variables. An improved version of MDS is expected to be nationally implemented in October 2010, while some anticipate possible disappointment as a consequence of its multipurpose use (Rahman and Applebaum 2009).

In the European Community, most member states have national quality standards for the care of elderly citizens. In some, they are legally binding while in others they are only recommendations and there is evidence that regional and local authorities have a greater degree of discretion in the standards they apply compared to health care (European Commission 2003). Overall, it seems that 'too little is being done in Europe, and where efforts are being made, it is unclear to what extent the information being collected is used to achieve better quality services' (Sorenson 2007a: 4).

Many challenges regarding quality evaluation and assurance in long-term care have been identified. They represent research and operational opportunities on the road to a better quality of life for all involved. Key aspects in need of further effort are the improvement of existing evaluation systems and methodologies so that they can function in integrated settings and serve a more comprehensive concept of quality of care and the exploring of ways of giving voice to stakeholders, whether users, users' carers or purchasers, because for them quality is what they perceive and not necessarily what others say exists.

In Portugal, quality assessment in long-term contexts is linked to recent reforms. Efforts are being made to set quality assurance and assessment systems at individual and organizational levels. The information available is still scarce, but the fact that several entities have begun to measure and report on the satisfaction of users of different types of long-term facilities in Portugal certainly deserves attention, even if results might be impaired by methodological issues.

Organizing for Long-term Care in Portugal

In Portugal, until recently there has been very little state provision of community care services, including long-term care, day centres and social services for the chronically ill, older people and other groups with special needs (Barros and Simões 2007), a situation with deep historical and socio-cultural roots.

Before the eighteenth century, hospitals and religious charities (*Misericórdias*) provided health care only to the poor. The development of public health services started in 1901 with a network of medical officers responsible for public health. In 1946, a mandatory social health insurance system was created – *Caixas de Previdência*. This system was financed by the contributions of employees and employers and provided out-of-hospital curative services, free at the point of use. After the democratic revolution in 1974, a process of nationalization began in health services. First, district and central hospitals owned by the religious charities were taken over by the government, as well as 2,000 medical units or health posts located throughout the country, previously operated under the social welfare system for the exclusive use of social welfare beneficiaries and their families. Public health services and health services provided by social welfare were brought together, leaving the general social security system to provide cash benefits and other social services, namely for the elderly and children. The National Health Service (NHS) was created in 1979 as a universal system, free at the point of use. Until then, the Portuguese state had left the responsibility for paying for health care to the individual patient and his/her family. Care of the poor was the responsibility of charity hospitals and the Department of Social Welfare was responsible for out-of-hospital care.

Regarding social care, traditionally the family assumed the first line of care, particularly in rural areas, but the situation is changing very quickly, mainly due to the high rate of Portuguese women in the labour market, demographic pressure, the increasingly complex nature of many cases and the epidemiological transition from predominantly acute to chronic conditions.

Some social services are provided in each region through the Ministry of Employment and Social Solidarity. However, IPSS (*Instituições Particulares de Solidariedade Social* – Non-Public Institutions for Social Solidarity), which are non-profit-making non-public institutions for social solidarity, and among them *Misericórdias*, have been the main providers of these services. They offer a number of social services, namely meals, laundry services and assistance in obtaining medication or health care. As family support has been decreasing, the state considers the IPSS a strategic part of the care system. Home care is expanding in Portugal and infrastructure to deliver support to the elderly has been developed in some regions through partnership between local government, regional health administrations and non-profit-making institutions.

Long-term care was identified as one of the gaps in Portuguese NHS coverage. Therefore, the National Network for Long-term Integrated Care (RNCCI) was created by Law no. 101/2006 within the scope of the Ministry of Health and the Ministry of Employment and Social Solidarity, based on existing institutions. It brings together teams providing long-term care, palliative action and social support with members coming from hospitals, health centres, local and district social security services, community services, local government and the Solidarity Network. Geographically, the network is organized at three levels of coordination, central, regional and local, aiming at improved governance and equity of access. Structurally, it is based on establishing protocols with existing institutions, designated according to the kind of services they provide as convalescence unit (*Unidade de Convalescença* – UC), medium-term and rehabilitation unit (*Unidade de Média Duração e Reabilitação* – UMDR), long-term and maintenance unit (*Unidade de Longa Duração e Manutenção* – ULDM), palliative care unit (*Unidade de Cuidados Paliativos* – UCP) and day care and autonomy promotion unit (*Unidade de Dia e de Promoção de Autonomia* – UDPA). Local coordination teams are located in specific health centres. Each team might coordinate the work of teams in several health centres in different but geographically close council areas. It is responsible for validating the reasons stated by the discharge team located in the acute care hospital for admission of each patient to the RNCCI and finding places in the appropriate unit of the network (figure 1).

One of the main, although possibly not stated, purposes of RNCCI is reducing costly acute care hospital cases and length of stay by substituting less costly care closer to the community. The network must be fully implemented within ten years (2006–16) but its final design will be the result of periodically assessed pilot experiences. Home care is supposed to be one important element in this network, but the conclusions of the report published in 2007 show there is a lot to be done in this particular field. During the pilot experiences, patients in need of primary home care were not being referred to the network and many of the patients referred are counting on their families and non-profit-making institutions' support also, to provide home social care. Another important conclusion is that the majority of patients discharged from the rehabilitation and palliative units of the network return to their homes or nursing homes, and that a significant percentage of these patients need home care (UMCCI July 2007). However, until now, this has been the weakest, least cared-for link of the network.

Structural Aspects and Attainment of Institutional Goals

The current situation of long-term care in Portugal still relies heavily on informal and privately funded care. In 2006, some 5,596 entities were identified as owners of social facilities, an increase of 5.1 per cent in relation to the

Figure 1

Organization of services in the different levels of care

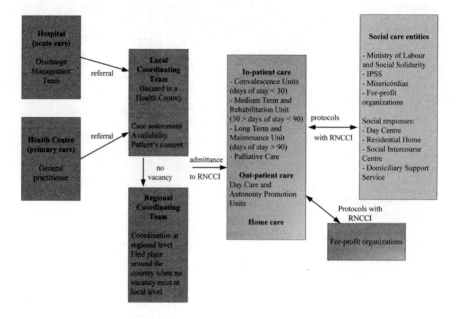

previous year (Ministério do Trabalho e da Solidariedade Social 2006). Of those, 72.7 per cent were non-profit-making organizations, with 65.9 per cent having the legal status of IPSS and 3.0 per cent of organizations comparable to IPSS. Detailed information is presented in table 1.

Regarding areas of intervention related to our working definition of long-term care, 51.1 per cent provided services to the elderly population, 5.4 per cent intervened in the rehabilitation and integration of handicapped people, 0.4 per cent were devoted to mental health and 1.9 per cent worked with other dependent persons. The number of social responses dedicated to the elderly population and the rehabilitation and integration of handicapped people increased by 46.4 and 43.4 per cent, respectively, from 1998 to 2006.

Provision of social care aimed at the needs of the elderly population was responsible for 36.1 per cent of the operating costs of the social network. Transformations occurring in Portuguese society, at the demographic and the family levels, lead to new types of intervention and to the adjustment of existing social responses. From 1998 to 2006, the Domiciliary Support Service (SAD – *Serviço de Apoio Domiciliário*) had the highest growth rate (75.5 per cent) in terms of number of facilities, followed by day centres (*centro de dia*) (40.6 per cent) and residential homes (*lar e residência*) for the elderly population (28.4 per cent). In the case of SAD, the capacity and the number of users more than doubled, corresponding to growth rates of 104 per cent and 109 per cent, respectively. The mean occupation rate of the services (day centre, residential

Table 1

Structural aspects related to social responses dedicated to dependent persons in 2006

Area of intervention, as % of the total number of facilities	
Services to the elderly population	51.1
Rehabilitation and integration of handicapped people	5.4
Mental health	0.4
Work with other dependent people	1.9
Growth in the number of social responses by public served, from 1998 to 2006 (%)	
Dedicated to the elderly population	46.4
Dedicated to the rehabilitation and integration of handicapped people	43.4
Cost, as % of the total cost of social responses	
Provision of social care to the elderly population	36.1
Growth in the number of social responses by type of intervention, from 1998 to 2006 (%)	
Domiciliary Support Service (SAD)	75.5
Day centres	40.6
Residential homes for the elderly population	28.4
Growth of SAD, from 1998 to 2006 (%)	
Capacity	104
Number of users	109
Occupation rate (%)	
Mean (day centre, residential home, SAD, social intercourse centre)	88.2
Residential home service – the highest	97.2
Coverage rate (%)	
National mean	11.1

Source: Ministério do Trabalho e da Solidariedade Social (2006).

home, Domiciliary Support Service and social intercourse centre) is 88.2 per cent. The occupation rate of the residential home service has always been the highest, attaining 97.2 per cent in 2006. Generically, supply is adequate to the ageing of the Portuguese population and follows geographical population distribution. In 2006, coverage rates for old people's homes, day-care centres and Domiciliary Support Service ranged from 20.1 to 48.9 per cent in 70 local council areas, while in 12 areas the maximum coverage rate was 5.6 per cent. The national mean was 11.1 per cent.

Regarding the RNCCI, a new monitoring report issued in August 2008 (UMCCI August 2008) states that a total number of 8,133 patients were referred to the network during the first semester of 2008, an increase of 103 per cent in relation to the period between November 2006 and December 2007 (see table 2).

Until the end of June 2008, the bodies with most protocols signed with the network were *Misericórdias* (61 per cent) and IPSS (16 per cent). At that time, only 11 per cent of the entities providing services to the network (such as UC and UCP) belonged to the National Health Service. The remaining contracts had been established with for-profit private institutions. In every type of unit, a mean 58 per cent of the referred users have been admitted. Of these, 30 per cent have been admitted to UMDR, 30 per cent to ULDM and 26 per cent to

Table 2

Structural aspects related to the functioning of the RNCCI in 2008

Patients referred during the first semester of 2008	
Absolute number	8133
Type of providers with protocols signed with the network, as % of the total	
Misericórdias	61
IPSS	16
Entities belonging to the NHS	11
For-profit private organizations	12
Admissions by type of unit, as % of the total of people admitted	
Medium term and rehabilitation unit (UMDR)	30
Long-term and maintenance unit (ULDM)	30
Convalescence unit (UC)	26
Demography of referred users	
Average age of women (years)	75
Average age of men (years)	72
Participation of women (%)	57
Prevalence of people with completed basic education (%)	72
Users receiving some kind of help by the time of admission (%)	58
Stroke as principal diagnosis (% of users)	32

Source: UMCCI (August 2008).

UC. Most admission proposals were generated by discharge management teams based at acute care hospitals. The average age of referred users is 75 for women and 72 for men; 57 per cent of those referred are women, 72 per cent have completed basic education and 58 per cent were receiving some kind of help at the time they were admitted to the health system. For 32 per cent of users, a stroke is referred to as the principal diagnosis.

During the first semester of 2008, 81 per cent of patients discharged from the RNCCI returned to their home. According to the monitoring report, most of them (67 per cent) did not have any identified need for integrated care support at the time of discharge. Achievement of therapeutic objectives was the reason for discharge in 70 per cent of cases. Occupation rate increased from 2007 to 2008 in all types of units except for those providing palliative care. The largest increase has been observed in convalescence units (from 65 to 89 per cent). In UMDR and ULDM, the occupation rate during the first semester of 2008 was nearly 100 per cent.

Regarding the financing and costs of the RNCCI, little has been disclosed, besides the division of costs forecast for 2008 between the health sector (80 per cent) and the social sector (20 per cent). This corresponds to implementation and operation of a total of 4,000 places in in-patient units, 15 places in day care and autonomy promotion units, 100 long-term integrated care teams, 74 discharge management teams, 14 intra-hospital teams for support in palliative care and 11 community teams for support in palliative care.

Access to the National Network for Long-term Integrated Care (RNCCI) is regulated by Article 31 of Law no. 101/2006 of 6 June. To be admitted, the person has to be in one or more of the following situations: transitory functional dependency due to a convalescence process or similar situation; prolonged functional dependency; being elderly with fragility criteria; severe incapacity, with strong psychosocial impact; severe illness, in an advanced or terminal phase. In practice, families able to take care of their relations who lose their independence still choose to take them home after discharge from hospital or to have them at home even in situations of great dependence. This situation is changing, not only due to the difficulty of ensuring care for these people at home, but also due to the growing availability of good-quality solutions allowed by admission to the RNCCI.

The National Health System is defined as universal, comprehensive and 'approximately free of charge' at the point of use by the Portuguese Constitution (1989 revision). Nevertheless, increasing co-payment and long waiting lists lead those with more resources to private hospitals and practices. The very poor and those with chronic diseases may be exempt from access tax to public services. Means-tested assistance with residential care provided by the public sector is available. Social services pay a proportion of residential costs depending upon income. The alternative is the nursing homes run by *Misericórdias* and other IPSS, which are of better quality and only request a nominal contribution from users and their families.

We have to bear in mind that this entire situation is currently changing rapidly, including the organization and responsibility of services, legislation ruling service provision, and financing models.

Quality, Suitability and Satisfaction from Users' Point of View

Information about the quality of services provided by the bodies under analysis and their users' satisfaction is scarce. Moreover, we could not find published studies reporting on results of evaluations conducted by external, independent entities. Therefore, the information reported here is based on results of evaluations conducted by or on behalf of the authorities supervising the networks and published in the Social Chart (Ministério do Trabalho e da Solidariedade Social 2005) and the RNCCI 2008 monitoring report (UMCCI 2008).

The Social Chart has been defined as an instrument aimed at presenting the network of social services and equipment tutored by the Ministry of Employment and Social Solidarity for Portuguese citizens (Ministério do Trabalho e da Solidariedade Social 2005). Part of the information is based on surveys involving personal interviews (Nicola 2007). In 2005, the procedure incorporated a module designed to collect some data about the quality of social responses and users' satisfaction, namely regarding the conditions offered by residential homes for the elderly (table 3).

Conditions of hygiene and human resources were perceived as of good quality, with more than 90 per cent of subjects classifying them as good or very good. Regarding the cost of co-financing by families, 60.7 per cent of interviewees considered it reasonable, while 26.4 per cent quoted it as expensive and 4.8 per cent very expensive. The cost of this service is considered as its

Table 3

Perceptions of conditions offered by residential homes for the elderly

Structural variables	
Hygiene	Good or very good for more than 90% of users
Human resources	Good or very good for more than 90% of users
Cost of co-financing by families	
Reasonable	for 60.7% of users
Expensive	for 26.4% of users
Very expensive	for 4.8% of users
Main problem	
Cost	for 50% of users
Lack of activities	for 21.4% of users
Few occupational workshops	for 21.4% of users
Level of satisfaction	
Very satisfied	75.4% of users
Reasons for having chosen the provider	
Proximity	for 33.3% of users
Suitability of services	for 25% of users
Others	for 25.4% of users
Service quality	for 16.3% of users

Source: Nicola (2007).

'main problem' by 50 per cent of users. Others have concentrated mostly on 'lack of activities' (21.4 per cent) and 'few occupational workshops' (21.4 per cent). Generically, 75.4 per cent of respondents have declared themselves very satisfied with the service provided. However, 'service quality' is not among the first reasons for having chosen the provider, with 16.3 per cent of answers. The main reasons are 'proximity to residence' (33.3 per cent), 'suitability of services' (25 per cent) and a quite significant 'others' (25.4 per cent).

Regarding the RNCCI, for the first time a report (UMCCI 2008) provides some information on the quality of service provided by the RNCCI entities, attesting gains in the autonomy of patients discharged from the network and a high level of user satisfaction with services, among other indicators. Reported results are based on activity data and on a survey of present and past users conducted between 1 January and 30 June 2008. The sample included 244 people using the network at the time of the survey and 188 former users. The average age of respondents is over 71 and the majority (56 per cent) are women. Almost 84 per cent have only basic education.

Only 17 respondents were referred by a health centre, while 92.3 per cent were referred by an acute care hospital. Most of the respondents (86 per cent) were living at their own residence at the time they were admitted to the health system and more than half (about 60 per cent) intend to return to their homes, while 21 per cent expect to go to live with family and 17.5 per cent say they will take up residence in a home for the elderly or an IPSS. About 88 per cent of interviewees say they feel accompanied in the long-term in-patient unit, be it by the family or by professionals.

Generically (86.7 per cent), users report having received sufficient information about their stay at the RNCCI unit. The level of satisfaction with several
features of the facilities is very high. On a scale from 1 (completely unsatisfied)
to 6 (completely satisfied), all get more than 4.7, with cleanliness, comfort and
gym receiving the highest score (5.1) and reading room the lowest (4.8).
Services and human resources (availability, sympathy, support) are also evaluated very satisfactorily by users. The lowest means were obtained for infor-
mative aspects (around 4.5) regarding the user's state of health, the functioning
of the unit and the reception orientation.

The RNCCI has defined an evaluation instrument denominated 'Bio-
psychosocial Evaluation'. The goal is to assess physical, functional, mental,
social and lifestyle conditions. The first evaluation shows significant gains in
the autonomy of users discharged from the network, with less incapacity, and
more independence. The RNCCI also has procedures in place to evaluate the
level at which contracts signed with service providers are being respected. The
first results stress the need for a strong improvement effort in the areas of
'management of care processes and information' and 'safety, facilities, equipment and instruments'.

Preferences Regarding Long-term Care in Portugal

Important information about the situation in Portugal is conveyed by a
Eurobarometer document (Eurobarometer 2007), reporting the results of a
survey conducted in 29 European countries between 25 May and 30 June 2007
(table 4). A total of 28,660 Europeans aged 15 and over were interviewed
regarding health, long-term care and care of the elderly.

Regarding becoming dependent because of a physical or mental
health condition, 50 per cent of the Portuguese feel this is likely or inevitable
(45 per cent for EU27) and 50 per cent declare they are worried about the idea
(54 per cent for EU27). However, only 18 per cent are saving or taking out
insurance to pay for future care (24 per cent for EU27) and 11 per cent have
discussed future needs with family or close friends (18 per cent for EU27).
Regarding assessment of home care services for dependent people in Portugal,
39 per cent classify it as good (42 per cent for EU27); 41 per cent find it easy
to reach and to gain access to (41 per cent for EU27) while 40 per cent find
availability difficult (25 per cent for EU27); 23 per cent find it affordable (27 per
cent for EU27) while 56 per cent find it unaffordable (32 per cent for EU27).
Regarding assessment of care services for dependent people provided by
nursing homes, 57 per cent of the Portuguese assess it as good (41 per cent for
EU27) while 32 per cent find it bad (23 per cent for EU27); 54 per cent find it
easy to reach and to gain access to (39 per cent for EU27) while 39 per cent
find availability difficult (28 per cent for EU27); only 23 per cent find it
affordable (21 per cent for EU27) while 72 per cent find it unaffordable (43 per
cent for EU27). Regarding the best care option for elderly parents, 44 per cent
of the Portuguese think they should live with one of their children (30 per cent
for EU27), while 20 per cent decide on public or private service providers
visiting their home and providing them with appropriate help and care (27 per
cent for EU27). Some 54 per cent think that professional care staff looking

Table 4

Perceptions on becoming dependent and preferences regarding long-term care in Portugal

	Portuguese (%)	EU (27) (%)
Becoming dependent		
Feel this is likely or inevitable	50	45
Worried about the idea	50	54
Saving or taking out insurance	18	24
Have discussed future needs with family or friends	11	18
Perceptions on quality of home-care services for dependent people		
Quality is good	39	42
Easy to reach or gain access to	41	41
Affordable	23	27
Unaffordable	56	32
Perceptions on quality of services provided by nursing homes		
Quality is good	57	41
Easy to reach or gain access to	54	39
Affordable	23	21
Unaffordable	72	43
Best care option for elderly patients		
Live with one of their children	44	30
Home visits by public or private service providers	20	27
Perceptions on care provided		
Care staff are highly committed and do an excellent job	54	59
Institutions offer insufficient standards of care	63	45
Professional care at home available at an affordable cost	29	31
Experience with long-term health care		
Have ever needed any regular help and long-term care	29	42
Help received was totally appropriate	64	58
Have never paid or expect to pay for it in the future	76	75
Expectations regarding being provided with the appropriate care		
Certain or probable	65	71
Assistance in own home by a relative	46	45
Assistance in own home by a professional care service	20	23
Assistance in own home by a person hired by them or by a relative	8	10
Assistance in the home of close family	3	4
Assistance in a nursing home	10	8
Preferences regarding future help and long-term care		
Assistance in own home by a relative	50	45
Assistance in own home by a professional care service	21	24
Assistance in own home by a person hired by them or by a relative	6	12
Assistance in the home of close family	4	5
Assistance in a nursing home	11	8
Beliefs regarding the financing of long-term care		
Finance their own care	43	48
Think they will not receive all the long-term care they will need for financial reasons	45	46

Source: Eurobarometer (2007).

after elderly people are highly committed and do an excellent job (59 per cent for EU27) but 63 per cent consider that institutions such as nursing homes offer insufficient standards of care (45 per cent for EU27). Only 29 per cent agree that professional care at home is available at an affordable cost (31 per cent for EU27).

Regarding experience with long-term health care, only 29 per cent of the interviewees have ever been in need of any regular help and long-term care over the last ten years either for themselves or someone close (42 per cent for EU27). Of these, 64 per cent assess the help received as totally appropriate (58 per cent for EU27) while 23 per cent find it only partly appropriate (31 per cent for EU27). When turning to paying for the long-term care of a parent, 76 per cent of the Portuguese have neither paid for it in the past nor are currently paying or expect to pay for it in the future (75 per cent for EU27). The Portuguese are less optimistic than Europeans in general regarding the probability of being provided with the appropriate help and long-term care in the future, as 65 per cent estimate this to be certain or probable against 71 per cent for EU27. Regarding ways of getting assistance if in need, 46 per cent of the Portuguese expect to be assisted in their own home by a relative (45 per cent for EU27), 20 per cent in their own home by a professional care service (23 per cent for EU27), 8 per cent in their own home by a personal carer hired by them or by a relative (10 per cent for EU27), 3 per cent in the home of one of their close family members (4 per cent for EU27) and 10 per cent in a long-term care institution (nursing home) (8 per cent for EU27).

Preferences follow a similar pattern: 50 per cent would prefer to be assisted in their own home by a relative (45 per cent for EU27), 21 per cent in their own home by a professional care service (24 per cent for EU27), 6 per cent in their own home by a personal carer hired by them or by a relative (12 per cent for EU27), 4 per cent in the home of one of their close family members (5 per cent for EU27) and 11 per cent in a long-term care institution (nursing home) (8 per cent for EU27). Regarding the financing of long-term care, 43 per cent of those interviewed believe they will finance their own care (48 per cent for EU27), while 45 per cent think they would not receive all the help and long-term care they would need for financial reasons (46 per cent for EU27), as it would be too expensive.

Discussion and Conclusion

In 2007 (Eurobarometer 2007), the Portuguese declared themselves worried about the idea of becoming dependent because of a physical or mental health condition but few had taken practical measures regarding such a situation. More than the quality of services provided at the patient's home or in nursing homes, the problematic aspects seem to be availability and affordability of long-term care services. Interestingly, the Portuguese are close to citizens of Southern and Eastern European countries when considering that an elderly father or mother not able to live alone should live with one of their children, and close to citizens of Northern and Western countries when stating that they would prefer to be looked after in their own home if they found themselves in such a situation. However, even in the latter situation the family is always perceived as the preferred caregiver. Meanwhile, long-term care in Portugal still relies heavily on informal and privately funded care.

To close the gap in NHS coverage, the state has created the RNCCI. In its first two years of activity, the programme has concentrated on establishing a network of units and teams aimed at providing institutionalized convalescence, rehabilitation, maintenance and palliative care. Home care is still residual in this context.

In Portugal, *Misericórdias* and IPSS are the entities historically and vocationally involved in long-term care from a perspective closer to the working definition adopted in this chapter. Maybe not surprisingly, they are playing a central role in the establishment of the RNCCI, being involved in 77 per cent of contracts signed with the network. At the same time, they seem to be adapting to the trends in Portuguese society, increasing the offer of places in homes for the elderly and home care services.

Up till now, the RNCCI has been handling mostly cases referred by acute care hospitals. This is part of a strategy designed to reduce the length of stay in expensive units but some friction inside the network is transferring the problem to subsequent levels of the chain. Continuous monitoring of the network and the experience gained will certainly be valuable in its adaptation to identified needs. A possible development might be a clear investment in home and community care, in line with the generalized restructuring of primary care currently taking place in Portugal.

Portugal is no exception among Mediterranean countries such as Spain and Italy regarding the traditionally important role played by informal care. However, socio-demographic and epidemiological changes seem to have led to very different state interventions. In Spain, several laws have extended the range of available services over the past decade (Rey 2009). The Law on the Promotion of Personal Autonomy and Care for People in a Situation of Dependency, approved in 2006 after many years of debate, created the Autonomy and Dependency Care System (SAAD). It also defines dependency, a condition classified in three degrees that mediate access to the system. The dependency care benefits, intended to cover all citizens in a situation of dependency by 2015, are tax-funded and may be either services or financial benefits but their social character is clearly assumed. In Portugal, as we have shown, the need for social care services only does not qualify a dependent person for admission to RNCCI. Interestingly, by 2006 the mean coverage rate of social care services in Portugal was 11.1 per cent (table 1), although with wide variations across the country, while in Spain public funding for essential services such as home help and residential care covered no more than 4 per cent of the population. Social care services are provided by both local authority and private-sector (mostly not-for-profit) providers and tend to be regulated by the autonomous governments (Comas-Herrera *et al.* 2006; Costa-Font and González 2008). Therefore, following the situation in the two countries in future years might prove valuable to understand the dynamics involved in such complex settings.

In Italy, state intervention regarding the care of the elderly population brought about new models of governance involving decentralization of the duty to plan and implement the health system to regional and local authorities and the use of the so-called Area Plans, which cover local social and health care projects and define the targets and activities of health and social care (Italian Ministry of Labour 2009). The Italian system relies strongly on private, home-based care, much of which is purchased in the grey economy, probably due to the existence of generous cash benefits (*indennità di accompagnamento*) that are not means-tested (Ungerson 2004) and the availability of immigrant carers (the so-called *badanti*). There are huge differences in the percentage of *indennità* users between the Italian regions, while attempts have been made by the national government to verify the real degree of disability of those benefiting from the scheme (see Costa-Font, this volume). In Portugal, the increase in the provision of home-based social care is one of the most important adjustments social care institutions are making to cope with the changes in Portuguese society and culture while the purchase of care work by families is residual. Therefore, the longitudinal study of the two arrangements might bring important knowledge regarding the long-term sustainability of these options, as well as the quality of outputs and the satisfaction of users.

In Portugal, information regarding the quality of services provided by all the bodies involved and the satisfaction of users is still scarce. Existing reports generally show very high levels of satisfaction with basic services provided and some impact on patients' quality of life. However, little is known about the methods used in these studies and conclusions have to be drawn with caution. Moreover, results from the Eurobarometer survey (Eurobarometer 2007) show that a significant percentage of Portuguese citizens have reservations about the quality of services provided by some of these entities.

Nevertheless, several instruments to assess performance have been adopted or are in the process of being introduced. The RNCCI has been particularly active in this regard, introducing the 'Bio-psychosocial Evaluation', an instrument with characteristics similar to the Minimum Data Set, implementing procedures to evaluate the level at which contracts signed with service providers are being respected and assessing users' satisfaction. Secondly, the Portuguese Institute for Social Security (ISS) has developed a quality model derived from the ISO 9001 standard and the EFQM (European Foundation for Quality Management) Model of Excellence and adapted to the different types of services provided by social care entities. The ISS has developed sets of materials intended to support quality improvement efforts that are now available over the web. The qualification of social services providers will result from quality audits conducted by independent certification bodies, but organizations are urged to adopt self-assessment and quality improvement practices. Unfortunately, little has been disclosed about the state of all these initiatives.

Above all, there is no independent information available on the interrelation between the technical quality of services provided, costs involved and satisfaction of stakeholders including patients, professionals and informal caregivers, citizens in general and society as a whole. Such a complex situation calls for a multidimensional approach to quality, focusing not only on the objective quality of the service provided, as measured by well-established and recognized standards, but also the quality the user perceives, the satisfaction she/he experiences and the financial effort required to provide a suitable level of service, according to a multifaceted perspective of service comprising access, affordability, technical quality, efficiency in using resources and a number of qualitative characteristics that include, among other things, the contribution to the user's quality of life, satisfaction and empowerment, compassion, empathy, transparency and ethical behaviour.

Acknowledgements

This work is partially funded by the European Commission in the context of EC-FP7-Homecare 222954.

References

Barros, P. and Simões, J. (2007), Portugal: health system review, *Health Systems in Transition*, 9, 5: 1–140.

Breckenkamp, J., Wiskow, C. and Laaser, U. (2007), Progress on quality management in the German health system: a long and winding road, *Health Research Policy and Systems*, 5, 7 (doi:10.1186/1478-4505-5-7).

Comas-Herrera, A., Wittenberg, R., Costa-Font, J., Gori, C., Maio, A. di, Patxot, C., Pickard, L., Pozzi A. and Rothgang, H. (2006), Future long-term care expenditure in Germany, Spain, Italy and the United Kingdom, *Ageing and Society*, 26: 285–302.

Costa-Font, J. and González, A. (2008), Long-term care reform in Spain, *Eurohealth*, 13, 1: 20–2.

Driest, P. (2006), Long-term care in Europe. In J. Hassink and M. Dijk (eds), *Farming for Health*, New York: Springer, pp. 101–6.

EC (2008), *Long-term Care in the European Union*, Brussels.

Eurobarometer (2007), Health and long-term care in the European Union, *Special Eurobarometer 283/Wave 67.3*, Brussels: European Commission.

European Commission (2003), *Joint Report by the Commission and the Council on Supporting National Strategies for the Future of Health Care and Care for the Elderly*, Brussels: Council of the European Union.

Italian Ministry of Labour (2009), Combining choice, quality and equity in social services, *Peer Review: Combining choice, quality and equity in social services – Denmark*.

Ministério do Trabalho e da Solidariedade Social (2005), *Carta Social: Rede de serviços e equipamentos. Um inquérito à qualidade, adequação e satisfação*, Lisbon.

Ministério do Trabalho e da Solidariedade Social (2006), *Carta Social: Rede de serviços e equipamentos*, Lisbon.

Mor, V. (2005), Improving the quality of long-term care with better information, *Milbank Quarterly*, 83, 3: 333–64.

Nicola, R. (2007), *Carta Social 2005: Rede de serviços e equipamentos – Um inquérito à qualidade, adequação e satisfação* (May), Direcção Geral de Estudos Estatística e Planeamento do Ministério do Trabalho e da Solidariedade Social, Lisbon.

OECD (2005), *Long-term Care for Older People*, Paris: OECD.

Rahman, A. N. and Applebaum, R. A. (2009), The nursing home minimum data set assessment instrument: manifest functions and unintended consequences –past, present, and future, *Gerontologist*, 49, 6: 727–35.

Rey, M. (2009), Combining choice, quality and equity in social services, *Peer Review: Combining choice, quality and equity in social services – Denmark*.

Satia, J. (1999), Achieving total quality management in public health systems, *Journal of Health Management*, 1, 2: 301–22.

Sorenson, C. (2007a), Quality measurement and assurance of long-term care for older people, *Euro Observer, The Health Policy Bulletin of the European Observatory on Health Systems and Policies*, 9, 2: 1–8.

Sorenson, C. (2007b), The US experience in long-term care quality measurement, *Euro Observer, The Health Policy Bulletin of the European Observatory on Health Systems and Policies*, 9, 2: 5–6.

UMCCI (July 2007), *Relatório de monitorização das experiências piloto da Rede Nacional de Cuidados Continuados Integrados*, Lisbon.

UMCCI (2008), *Relatório semestral de monitorização do desenvolvimento da Rede Nacional de Cuidados Continuados Integrados em 2008*, Lisbon.

UMCCI (August 2008), *Relatório semestral de monitorização do desenvolvimento da Rede Nacional de Cuidados Continuados Integrados em 2008*, Lisbon.

Ungerson, C. (2004), Whose empowerment and independence? A cross-national perspective on 'cash for care' schemes, *Ageing and Society*, 24, 2: 189–212.

World Health Organization (2007), *Financing Long-term Care Programmes in Health Systems*, Discussion paper no. 6, Geneva: WHO.

Index